T0143652

# BASIC HEALTH
# PUBLICATIONS
## USER'S GUIDE

# TO
# THYROID
# DISORDERS

*Natural Ways to Keep
Your Body from
Dragging You
Down.*

## KATHLEEN BARNES
### JACK CHALLEM Series Editor

Series Editor: Jack Challem
Editor: Susan Andrews
Typesetter: Gary A. Rosenberg
Series Cover Designer: Mike Stromberg

Basic Health Publications User's Guides are published by Basic Health Publications, Inc.

# CONTENTS

# INTRODUCTION

**A** tiny butterfly-shaped gland that straddles your windpipe and weighs less than an ounce sends signals to every one of the trillions of cells in your body billions of times every single day. It governs every cellular and bodily function. Without it, you'd wind down like a child's toy. Eventually, you would die.

Many experts believe thyroid disease is the most underdiagnosed illness in America. A paper published in the *Journal of the American Medical Association* (JAMA) nearly sixty years ago asserted that low thyroid function is the most common disease of those who enter the doctor's office—and it's the diagnosis most doctors most often miss. While we have more high tech tools available for diagnosis today than we did in the 1950s, long-time sufferers of debilitating fatigue, susceptibility to cold temperatures, intractable weight gain, shortness of breath, and dozens of other widely diverse symptoms, find little more relief today than their grandparents did in country doctors' offices two generations ago.

In this book, you'll learn that a straightforward diagnosis of hypothyroidism is difficult to obtain. A diagnosis of subclinical hypothyroidism (under-the-radar low thyroid function that is not confirmed by tests) is even more difficult to obtain, unless you know how to find a doctor who is willing to prescribe thyroid medication based on symptoms rather than lab tests.

If you've grappled with the hash of symptoms that can indicate hypothyroidism (and several other clinical conditions), you may have been subjected to accusations that you are lazy, a hypochondriac, PMS-ing, or perhaps even a little mentally unbalanced. Your problem may be compounded by the possibility that the tendency to hypothyroidism may have been present in your family for generations.

Recent statistics show that up to 10 percent of Americans have thyroid disease or will develop it. As of this writing, more than 13 million Americans have been diagnosed with thyroid deficiency; approximately 50 percent of sufferers are not diagnosed.

In fact, the late Dr. Broda Barnes, a pioneer in the study of thyroid malfunction, estimated that up to 40 percent of all Americans have some degree of thyroid disorder.

Women are five to eight times more likely to have thyroid deficiency for a number of reasons, among them the likelihood there is an as yet-undiscovered female hormonal component to this complex disease.

"Even a slight deficiency in thyroid hormone can cause an incredible number and variety of sabotaging physical, emotional, and mental symptoms," writes Stephen Langer, M.D., in *Solved: The Riddle of Illness.*

Calling low thyroid function an "undeclared epidemic," Richard Shames, M.D., and Karilee Halo Shames, Ph.D., R.N., authors of *Thyroid Power*, pinpoint the problem precisely: "Although extremely common, low thyroid is largely an unsuspected illness. Even when suspected, it is frequently undiagnosed. When it is diagnosed, it often goes untreated. When it is treated, it is seldom treated optimally."

Although this book will primarily address hypothyroidism, which is by far the most common form of thyroid dysfunction, other forms of thyroid and glandular malfunction can wreak equal havoc with your life, and I'll address them, too. Hyperthyroidism (overactive thyroid), Hashimoto's thyroiditis (an autoimmune form of hypothyroidism), and Graves' disease (autoimmune overactive thyroid) will be addressed in Chapter 6, and I'll discuss the link between hypothyroidism and adrenal imbalance in Chapter 5.

This book will present thyroid dysfunction in simple terms and hopefully help you understand the complexities of thyroid function and malfunction so you can navigate the stormy seas of the modern medicine, dispel myths about natural treatments perpetuated by the medical profession, and find a diagnosis and correct treatment.

# CHAPTER 1

# THE BASIC SCIENCE

**M**ost of us are aware that the thyroid secretes a variety of hormones. What you may not realize is that these hormones affect virtually every one of the trillions of cells in your body and every single body function. Without these hormones, you cannot survive in the long term.

The late Broda Barnes, M.D., pioneer of thyroid research and treatment, once wrote about his participation in a medical school experiment: "Students were shocked at the rapid deterioration of a small rabbit after removal of its thyroid. Previously warm at room temperatures, active, and alert, the animal now shivered with cold, moved in slow motion, drugged with fatigue—as if old and feeble. Its skin was scaly, its mucous membranes were infected—particularly in the respiratory system—and its heartbeat and muscles were weak."

Sound familiar? The thyroid has been likened to a gas pedal, producing hormones that fuel your entire body. To stretch out the metaphor to the breaking point, when you have a lead foot and push on the gas pedal too hard for too long, your car first runs out of gas and eventually breaks down, usually at the most inconvenient time. That's what's happening when the thyroid's hormone production begins to deteriorate—there's simply been too much pressure on the little gland for too long.

## Thyroid Function 101

Your thyroid produces several types of hormones. The two most important are T3 (triiodothyronine) and T4 (thyroxine). These two help get oxygen

**Triidothyronine (T3)**
*The biologically active hormone; comprises 20 percent of thyroid hormone produced by your body; of the two, it is the stronger hormone.*

into your cells, and the oxygen burns calories. In other words, they control your metabolism. Imagine what would happen if there were no oxygen in your cells and no calories burning. It might look very much like Dr. Barnes' poor rabbit—or like you, if you're suffering from hypothyroidism. The cells of the thyroid gland are the only ones in your body capable of using iodine—and with the help of tyrosine molecules, iodine helps your body form T3 and T4. In fact, the "3" and "4" in these two hormones refers to the number of iodine molecules in each molecule of thyroid hormone.

**Thyroxine (T4)**
*The most plentiful thyroid hormone; it constitutes about 80 percent of thyroid hormone produced by your body, and is converted to T3 by the liver and hypothalamus.*

A healthy thyroid produces about 80 percent T4 and 20 percent T3, even though T3 has four times the hormone strength of T4. The additional T3 your body needs is converted from T4 in other organs, including the liver and the hypothalamus, a part of your brain. The hypothalamus plays another important function: It regulates the thyroid's production of T3 and T4 by telling the pituitary gland to release TSH or thyroid-stimulating hormone.

In their book *Thyroid Power*, Drs. Richard and Karilee Shames call thyroid "a tiny but powerful throttle mechanism, because the energy hormone it produces (T3) acts like a gas pedal for the rest of the body." But when the production or circulation of T3 and T4 are out of whack, the hypothalamus and pituitary try to correct the shortfall by sending out more TSH, asking for more production of the essential thyroid hormones.

## Causes of Thyroid Malfunction

Thyroid malfunction is caused by a wide variety of

factors, including the chronic stress of the fast-paced life most of us live.

If your energy levels have flagged, it can be due to any of the following:

- The thyroid can't make enough T4.

- The T4 is not being converted to its active form, T3.

- The adrenal glands have become too weak to handle the body's normal rate of metabolism, so they go on strike and force a slowdown in energy production.

- The enzymes (cellular machinery) that makes ATP (adenosine-triphosphate), the cell's major energy carrier, may be held back due to chemical interference such as toxins, lack of needed nutrients, or breakdown due to autoimmune disease or viral damage.

- Imbalances in hormones such as estrogen, progesterone, and testosterone can affect energy production.

- Starvation leads to energy slowdown, which explains why it's not good to fast for extended periods of time.

Since you now know that every cell of your body needs thyroid hormone to function properly, it stands to reason that when thyroid function is impaired, nothing in your body is functioning at an optimal level.

Some clinical causes of hypothyroidism include surgical removal of the thyroid for various reasons, including cancer; radioactive iodine treatment for hyperthyroidism or Graves' disease that essentially destroys the thyroid; and radiation treatment to the head, neck, or chest for any reason.

## Smoking and Other Factors Affecting Hypothyroidism

Smoking has been strongly associated with hypothyroidism. A 1995 Swiss study published in the *New England Journal of Medicine* states that a multitude of substances in tobacco smoke decrease the secretion of thyroid hormones and lessen overall thyroid function.

Certain medications such as lithium (sometimes used for bipolar disorder), amiodarone (a heart drug), estrogen, and sulfa drugs can cause hypothyroidism.

However, some of the preeminent experts, like Dr. Jacob Teitelbaum, author of *From Fatigued to Fantastic,* think immune system dysfunction is a factor in many, if not most, cases of hypothyroidism and that our increasing exposure to toxins in our environment and in our food supply has fueled this autoimmune type of thyroiditis.

## Iodine

Most people have some idea that iodine is connected to thyroid disorders. This is true, since the thyroid gland is the only part of the human body that processes dietary iodine. Thyroid problems have long been linked to iodine deficiency. Iodine was added to salt and bread manufactured in the United States after early twenthieth-century epidemiological reports showed a "Midwest Goiter Belt" where there was an unusually large rate of enlarged thyroids.

In some countries, there is a shortfall of dietary iodine and in other areas, overconsumption of dietary iodine. Too much or too little iodine can cause the thyroid confusion that leads to thyroid exhaustion and an inability to produce the T3 and T4 necessary to maintain proper metabolism and energy levels.

Since we are such a salt- and bread-loving nation, it would stand to reason that Americans are iodine sufficient, but that is the subject of controversy.

### Iodine Deficiency?

The first National Health and Nutrition Examination

Survey (NHANES I), which took place between 1971and 1974, found that just 2.6 percent of U.S. citizens had iodine deficiency. The follow-up NHANES III survey, conducted between 1988 and 1994, found that 11.7 percent were iodine deficient.

A 1998 article published in the *Journal of Clinical Endocrinology and Metabolism* said that the percentage of Americans with low intake of iodine more than quadrupled between 1978 and 1998. Researchers did not pinpoint a cause for this increase, but suggest that reduced salt in the diet, plus a reduction in the use of iodine as a food ingredient may be responsible.

There is great controversy about iodine's role in the escalating rate of hypothyroidism. Some practitioners think most hypothyroid patients should take iodine or a high-iodine herb like kelp or bladderwrack. Others suggest moderate doses in the 100-to-150 microgram range (this is the government's recommended range as well) are sufficient and may even be excessive for some patients. Still others recommend megadoses.

However, before pursuing this course, you can ask for an iodine-loading test in which a large dose of iodine is given and then recovered in the urine to discover how much is being retained by your body. This test is not well known or widely used, but it can be very helpful, according to Ron Hunninghake, M.D., a specialist in natural thyroid treatment from Wichita, Kansas.

### The Minimalist Camp

Many people think consuming more iodine or even taking supplemental iodine is a good way to "jump start" an underactive thyroid. Instead, they may actually be further irritating an already challenged thyroid, causing additional problems, according to another school of thought.

Dr. Shames, coauthor of *Feeling Fat, Fuzzy or Frazzled?*, for example, says the iodine question is a difficult one. In many countries, too little iodine is a major health issue, causing infertility, miscarriages, birth defects, goiters, and mental retardation. On the other hand, as Dr. Shames notes, the industrialized world is finding that *excessive* iodine intake has become a problem.

"Iodine excess in genetically thyroid-sensitive people causes increased autoimmune difficulty. This autoimmune problem is separate from the high-or-low iodine problem but these issues overlap and influence each other," say Dr. Shames and his wife, Karilee, in *Feeling Fat, Fuzzy or Frazzled*?

According to Dr. Shames, high doses of iodine as recommended by some practitioners may be helpful for people and assist in breast and immune health as well, yet he recommends against this type of therapy because "In this country, I think hypothyroidism has little to do with iodine and more to do with autoimmune dysfunction. At the present time, I'm not doing the iodine thing. I don't recommend immediately upping the iodine intake if you're getting 100–150 micrograms a day."

Another part of the double-edged sword on the issue of iodine is that excess iodine can cause severe flare-ups in autoimmune thyroid disorders like Hashimoto's disease, he says. High amounts of iodine concentrate in the thyroid increase levels of a prehormone or hormone precursor called thyroglobulin, which in turn can trigger an autoimmune response, he concludes, urging caution in the use of iodine.

### The Middle Road

Mary Shomon, a patient advocate and author of *Living Well with Hypothyroidism*, also recommends caution; she says some patients get better with iodine and others get worse.

"If, like many patients, you decide on your own to try kelp, iodine, or one of the many thyroid-supporting supplements (almost all of them contain fairly large amounts of iodine or kelp), to see if they can help you, be aware of the risks. A percentage of patients is very sensitive to iodine/kelp supplementation, and find that it aggravates their thyroid problem," she says, affirming the link between iodine and autoimmune thyroiditis flare-ups.

### The Megadose Camp

Dr. Hunninghake notes that the Japanese consume an average 12 milligrams of iodine a day in their traditional diet, which is heavy on seafood and sea vegetables. That's 125 times the amount the American government's recommends! The *Merck Manual* says that in some parts of the world, notably Japan, the typical diet can exceed 50 milligrams of iodine a day, with no higher rate of thyroid dysfunction there than elsewhere.

Dr. Hunninghake has used the iodine loading test and given doses similar to those in the Japanese diet. He recommends iodine in a product called Iodoral. Each tablet contains 5 milligrams of iodine and 7.5 milligrams of potassium iodide, to help in the uptake of the iodine.

He bases his recommendation on the work of David Brownstein, M.D., a Michigan holistic thyroid practitioner and the author of *Iodine, Why You Need It, Why You Can't Live Without It*, who recommends megadoses of iodine to address resistant thyroid problems. Dr. Hunninghake says he has had excellent results using Brownstein's methods with about fifty hypothyroid patients who tested for low iodine.

Other possible causes of hypothyroidism are discussed below.

## Fluoride

Fluoride, the chemical waste product of the aluminum, steel, and fertilizer industries, has been a known thyroid inhibitor since 1854; yet, in the hopes of preventing tooth decay, officials began adding it to municipal water supplies in the 1950s. This decision was based on research from a decade earlier that has now been called into question. Fluoride is still added to the water supplies in 60 percent of American cities.

Fluoride is also found in many toothpastes and mouthwashes, in soft drinks and processed foods; it even occurs naturally in some fruits and vegetables. Experts now estimate we are taking in eight times the recommended levels of fluoride! Fluoride has long been a standard treatment for hyperthyroidism, so it stands to reason that if you get more fluoride, your thyroid function will slow even more.

## Environmental Pollutants in Drinking Water

Other pollutants in drinking water, some of them even present in well water, can cause thyroid problems. Among them are resorcinol, perchlorate, dihydroxy-benzoic acids, methylanthracene, and bromoform. These known thyroid inhibitors are waste products of various types of mining and plastic manufacturing, and even include pollutants accumulated when rural rivers and streams fill up with organic matter and fertilizer runoff.

## Goitrogenic Foods

Excess consumption of raw cruciferous vegetables (broccoli, cauliflower, Brussels sprouts) plus an overfondness for turnips, mustard greens, spinach, and rutabagas can slow thyroid function. These foods are known as goitrogens because eating large amounts of them can result in goiters. Other goitrogens include: walnuts, almonds, sorghum, peanuts,

---

### Beware of Plastic Containers

The same chemicals involved in plastics manufacturing that can pollute water supplies can transfer into water when it's stored in plastic containers. Avoid drinking bottled water from plastic containers, and if you do, never increase your exposure to degrading plastic components by re-using the same container more than twice.

pine nuts, millet, and cassava. While all of these foods are healthy and moderate consumption of them is good for you, it's not a good idea to eat them by the pound. Cooking neutralizes most goitrogens, so if you want to eat them, be sure they are cooked.

We'll take a closer look at food and thyroid in Chapter 9.

## Soy Products

This is an area of great controversy in the medical community. Many vegetarians consume several servings of various soy products daily as a major source of protein.

Several studies suggest a link between heavy soy consumption and thyroid dysfunction. Soy iso-flavones appear to elevate T4 without modifying T3, resulting in weight gain and impaired thyroid function.

## Certain Drugs and Chemicals

Prednisone, sulfa drugs, antidiabetic agents, birth control pills, and hormone-replacement therapies containing estrogen have all been implicated in lowering thyroid function. Some cough medicines, antidepressants, corticosteroids, and even aspirin can also slow thyroid hormone availability. Cigarette smoke, whether you're a smoker or are getting sec-ondhand smoke, is also a factor.

## Exposure to Radiation

Unless you live near the site of a nuclear power plant release, or you have had radiation treatments for cancer, it's unlikely that you have received enough radiation to affect thyroid function.

The 1986 Chernobyl nuclear power–plant acci-dent in the former Soviet Union, caused a large number of malfunctioning thyroids and a tenfold increase in thyroid cancers in a dozen countries when a radioactive iodine-131 gas cloud spread over the region. However, people living near the

Japanese Tokaimura nuclear-power plant that released radiation in 1999 were immediately given an inexpensive remedy—potassium iodide pills that prevent the thyroid from absorbing the radiation. The pills must be taken within twenty-four hours of exposure and cost less than ten cents each. If you live near a nuclear power plant and think you are at risk, keep a bottle of potassium iodide on hand.

## Immune System Malfunction

Drs. Shames—and many other experts—theorize that hypothyroidism is actually an autoimmune disease. "It turns out that the cause of virtually all cases of low thyroid is not so much a faulty thyroid gland as it is an overzealous immune system. As strange as it may seem, common low thyroid is a mild immune system illness in which the immune system wrongly attacks the innocent thyroid gland. The illness is called Hashimoto's thyroiditis, in honor of the Japanese doctor who first identified it," they wrote in *Thyroid Power.* Hashimoto's disease is an insidious form of hypothyroidism because its symptoms usually have a slow onset and so can go unaddressed for years.

In a toxic world replete with environmental toxins, chemical additives in food, pseudo-hormones, emotional and mental stress, our immune systems desperately seek to fight off the toxic effects by churning out antibodies that attack our own glands and hormones. The result is an inflamed thyroid incapable of producing the necessary amounts of T3 and T4 to keep our bodies functioning optimally.

# CHAPTER 2

# A COMPLEX LIST
# OF SYMPTOMS

**D**ozens of symptoms have been associated with hypothyroidism, and while all of them seem disconnected, they all potentially signal other types of health problems. You might experience several of these symptoms or only one or two. You might experience symptoms that seem contradictory, such as weight gain and diminished appetite or feeling cold and then hot.

This makes hypothyroidism difficult to diagnose, especially when doctors are reluctant to treat sub-clinical hypothyroidism. We'll talk more about that in Chapter 3, but when you see the laundry list of symptoms that may suggest your thyroid is under-active, you'll begin to get an idea of how pervasive this dysfunction can be.

## The Most Common Symptoms

The most common symptoms of hypothyroidism are intractable weight gain, fatigue, and cold intolerance, but the presence or absence of one of these is not sufficient either to arrive at or rule out a diagnosis. For some, the symptoms are extremely mild and for others, they are severe. However, the severity of symptoms does not seem to be an indicator of the seriousness of the thyroid deficiency.

Mary Shomon, author of *Living Well with Hypothyroidism*, says the symptoms of hypothyroidism usually become more pronounced as the TSH levels rise. "The number and severity of symptoms appears to be unique with each individual. Some people suffer terribly at a TSH of 15. Others have written to me about "not feeling quite up to par," only to discover they have a TSH of over 200." The Thyroid Foundation of America lists just over a dozen symptoms of hypothyroidism, "This list is just the tiniest tip of a very deep and very large iceberg," says Shomon.

## The Longer List

This list of symptoms runs roughly from most common to least common:

### Weight and Appetite

Weight gain
Weight loss
Diminished appetite
Increased appetite
Carbohydrate cravings

Food allergies and
   sensitivities
General bloating
Facial bloating

### Energy

Exhaustion
Weakness
Lethargy

Excessive sleeping
Waking up
   unrefreshed

### Body Temperature

Cold intolerance,
   particularly hands
   and feet

Low morning basal
   body temperature
Hot-cold temperature
   swings

### Hair and Nails

Dry, brittle hair
Hair loss
Loss of eyelashes

Loss of outer one-third
   of eyebrows
Thin, brittle nails

### Skin

Dry, itchy skin
Thickening of skin

Pimples, blackheads
Little or no perspiration

### Digestion

Constipation (may not respond to increased
   dietary fiber)

### Joints, Muscles, Nerves

Painful and sensitive
Carpal tunnel syndrome
Tendonitis
Tarsal tunnel syndrome (toes)
Plantar fasciitis

### Mental Function

Brain fog
Depression
Restlessness
Mood swings
Forgetfulness
Anxiety
Irritability

### Sex Drive

Decreased interest in sex
Difficulty reaching orgasm

### Vital Signs

Slow pulse
Heart palpitations
Low blood pressure
Unexplained high cholesterol
Drug-resistant high cholesterol

### Breathing

Sleep apnea
Snoring
Shortness of breath
Tightness in chest
Feeling of needing to yawn to get sufficient oxygen

### Allergies

Suddenly developing
Old allergies growing worse

### Eyes

Bulging eyes
Gritty, dry eyes
Light sensitivity
Tics that may result in headaches

### Women's Health Problems

Irregular menstrual periods
Heavy menstrual flow
Infertility
Miscarriage

### Men's Health Problems
Impotence

### Neck and Throat
Swelling in the neck

Feeling of pressure
around neck

### Hearing
Tinnitus (ringing in ears)

### Other Symptoms
Low, husky voice in
women
Dizziness,
lightheadedness
Headache

Increased numbers
of infections and
susceptibility to
colds and flu
Anemia

The above list contains more than seventy symptoms of hypothyroidism, but if you search hard you might be able to double the length of the list. It's a laundry list that's all over the map. You may experience just one or two or a dozen or more symptoms. You may barely be able to move or you may lead a relatively full life. With this many strange things going on in your body, it's no wonder doctors accuse hypothyroidism sufferers of being hypochondriacs or having a few screws loose!

## Other Possible Causes
There are many other health conditions that can cause similar symptoms. A few come readily to mind: perimenopause (pre-menopause), chronic yeast overgrowth, fibromyalgia, chronic fatigue syndrome, and Epstein-Barr syndrome.

It's easy to determine if you are in perimenopause with a panel of hormone tests. There is an apparent hormonal link between hypothyroidism and perimenopause that science has not yet pinpointed, but the two conditions often exist side by side.

Chronic candida-yeast overgrowth is worth investigating, although there are no definitive tests to determine if yeast is causing the symptoms. The best way to address yeast overgrowth is by strict adherence to a yeast-fighting diet that eliminates all sugars, most grains, and fruit and fermented products for three weeks or more and simultaneously journaling your symptoms to track your progress. Supplements can be helpful and some prescription drugs may even be required to get the yeast overgrowth under control.

**Candidiasis**
*A yeast infection, caused by the fungus Candida albicans, which can be found in the intestines, and can contribute to weight gain.*

Fibromyalgia and its kissing cousin, chronic fatigue syndrome, are believed to have an autoimmune component and are usually treated with dietary changes, supplementation, and a moderate exercise program.

Finally, Epstein-Barr, another close cousin of chronic fatigue, is a member of the herpes virus family that causes mononucleosis. Some herbal and supplemental treatments may be helpful and prescription antiherpes drugs are sometimes necessary.

**Chronic Fatigue Syndrome**
*Severe fatigue that lasts six months or more and is not explained by any other medical conditions. Symptoms include impaired concentration, sore throat, tender lymph nodes, muscle pain, joint pain, headaches, unrefreshing sleep, and extreme fatigue after exercise.*

All of these other possible causes for your symptoms are difficult to diagnose and are likely to lead you onto the medical merry-go-round, running from doctor to doctor in search of a diagnosis. Of all of these possibilities, hypothyroidism is the most easily treatable and you can find relief from these symptoms in just a few weeks.

## A Gordian Knot

Hypothyroidism often goes hand in hand with one of these or other low-energy diseases. Drs. Richard

and Karilee Shames write in *Thyroid Power:* "Coex-
istent low thyroid can worsen any other illness,
and—interestingly enough—the opposite is also
true. To achieve lasting improvement, you may have
to treat more than one condition at a time. It is crit-
ical that you obtain a full and complete diagnosis
and treat in the appropriate order all conditions that
may be contributing to your health dilemma."

Conversely, most of us can identify with at least
some of the symptoms on this lengthy list I've cited
above. Just because you're tired, or having difficulty losing weight, or you're constipated, doesn't in
any way mean you have an underactive thyroid.
These symptoms can indicate many disparate problems—or no real problem at all.

## Symptoms of Hypothyroidism in Children

Hypothyroidism can cause many of the same symptoms in children as are manifested in adults, so if
your child is showing any of the symptoms in the list
on pages 16–17, have his or her thyroid checked.

In addition, infants' symptoms may include poor
muscle tone; poor eating habits; thick coarse hair
growing low on forehead; a large, soft spot on the
head; prolonged jaundice; a herniated naval; and
little or no growth. Children's hypothyroidism is
often manifested in failure to grow, but the condition can also cause delayed puberty and problems
that may be diagnosed as attention-deficit disorder.
Since hypothyroidism has a genetic component,
your child is more at risk if you have the disease or
if any member of your family has it.

# CHAPTER 3

# DIAGNOSIS

**D**iagnosis is probably the most difficult part of having thyroid disease. Even if doctors were able to spend an hour with each patient, it would be difficult to diagnose thyroid disease because of its myriad symptoms and because of its ability to fly under the radar of screening tests.

In the real world, we get something like six to eight minutes of "face time" with our doctors. One study says doctors "tune out" their patients after just seven seconds!

When you think of the overwhelming list of symptoms in Chapter 2 and the complexity of thyroid problems, it's not surprising that so many patients are misdiagnosed, underdiagnosed, or never diagnosed at all. Patient advocate Mary Shomon aptly describes the diagnostic dilemma in her book, *The Thyroid Diet:* "You may find your doctor isn't willing to test your thyroid. Sometimes it's because the test was *your* idea, which can threaten a doctor's ego or sense of control. Or your doctor may be afraid that you want thyroid drugs as weight-loss aids. Some HMO doctors face restrictions or financial disincentives to order laboratory tests. Finally, some doctors are simply not particularly aware of or informed about thyroid disease."

## A Sad Tale

Doctors may tell you you're too young to have thyroid disease, or that they can tell by looking at you that you don't have a thyroid problem, or that they can't feel anything wrong by palpitating your thyroid, or even that it's impossible for you to have thyroid disease because you're male.

It's frustrating and even humiliating to be accused of being lazy, undisciplined, old, hypochondriacal, depressed, and/or crazy when you have an endocrine dysfunction.

Some doctors have their bank balances in mind when they decline to order tests. This may be because managed care, particularly HMOs, restricts fees dramatically and may even provide incentives to physicians for not ordering laboratory tests, not treating patients, and not referring them to specialists. As Dr. Jacob Teitelbaum notes in his book, *From Fatigued to Fantastic,* these types of doctors simply "hope you'll go away."

The bottom line, says endocrinologist Ron Hunninghake, M.D., is how the patient feels. "Ninety-five percent of doctors aren't treating the patient based on how he or she feels. They treat based on what the lab tests say. The patient might as well drive up to the window, stick his arm out and get a blood draw and get test results," says Dr. Hunninghake. He continues, "My point is that doctors aren't paying attention to what's going on with the patient. They're completely focused on lab tests, so at the end of the day, they base everything on what the lab says and not what the patient says."

## Countering Medical Resistance

If you encounter such medical resistance or downright ignorance, I strongly recommend that you seek medical help elsewhere.

If you have no options, here are some suggestions from Mary Shomon, author of *The Thyroid Diet:*

• Be persistent. Ask for a test. Ask again and again.

• Show your doctor articles about hypothyroidism that reflect your symptoms.

• Bring a detailed symptom list to your appointment, including dates, and ask your doctor to read it, sign it and include it in your chart. Keep a signed copy for yourself.

- Send a copy of your signed symptoms list to your insurance company's ombudsman or consumer liaison with a request that testing be approved.

- Write a letter to your health insurance company explaining your request to be tested for thyroid disease and your symptoms, and cite your doctor's refusal to order tests. Ask your doctor to sign the letter, give you a signed copy, and place another copy in your chart. Send the signed copy to your insurer to argue for testing or referral to another doctor or a specialist.

It may be difficult to ask a doctor to document a refusal to order tests, but physicians' fears of malpractice suits or mismanagement charges are great, and it's likely you will win if you just keep fighting, says Shomon. Dr. Teitelbaum suggests you may even have to engage the services of a lawyer to persuade a recalcitrant insurance company to give you the treatment to which you are entitled. Let's hope that's not the case, but be prepared to fight if need be. With all these hassles, ignorance and resistance, it's no surprise that patients trek from doctor to doctor, sometime for years, before they get relief. Sadly, some never do get a diagnosis that will help them.

### Self-Diagnosis the Easy Way

Thyroid pioneer Dr. Broda Barnes spent his medical career studying the effects of thyroid dysfunction. Beginning in the early 1930s, he studied thousands of patients and came to three groundbreaking conclusions that remain true today:

1. No less than 40 percent of the adult population of the United States suffers from hypothyroidism.

2. The vast majority of people with low thyroid function also have low basal body temperatures.

3. Low basal body temperatures are the best indica-

tors of hypothyroidism even when clinical testing shows "normal" thyroid function.

The Barnes Basal Temperature Test is an extremely simple at-home test that anyone can perform. The only equipment you'll need is an ordinary mercury oral thermometer.

## Barnes Basal Body Temperature Test

Here's how to do the test:

- Shake down the thermometer before you go to sleep and place it on your bedside table.

- Immediately upon awakening, without getting out of bed, place the thermometer in your armpit.

- Lie quietly and keep the thermometer in place for at least ten minutes.

- Take your reading at the same time every day for the next four days. If you are a woman still in your menstrual years, begin on the third day of your period. Men and non-menstruating women can take the tests any time of the month.

If your reading is consistently below 97.8 degrees, it's likely you have hypothyroidism.

If your Barnes Body Temperature Test suggests low thyroid function and you have as few as one or two of the symptoms described in Chapter 2, you should see a doctor and pursue further testing and treatment. For some enlightened practitioners, low body temperature is sufficient to begin a low dosage of thyroid hormone to see if you get relief from your symptoms.

## Are Blood Tests Worthwhile?

Dr. Sanford Siegel, author of *Is Your Thyroid Making You Fat?*, questions the value of blood tests for a variety of reasons, including common human errors in laboratories and inaccurate results when a patient is already taking some thyroid hormones or supplements. Dr. Siegel says tests may not define the real problem:

"The real problem may be quite remote from any of (the values yielded by lab tests). Is the amount of thyroid hormone circulating in the blood really all that important? It is recognized that the hormone does its work only when it reaches the cells that will be affected by it. Is it possible that cells in one person react differently from those in another? Could there be a defect not in the thyroid or its hormones, but in other parts of the body so that they don't take proper advantage of the hormone?"

Siegel relies on his own observations of the patient, what the patient tells him, and the Barnes Basal Body Temperature Test to help him begin the diagnostic process. Dr. Teitelbaum agrees. His theory about the inaccuracy of blood tests is based on studies that show TSH levels have little relationship to the actual amounts of T4 available to your cells.

## TSH: Myth and Reality

Imagine your thyroid gland as a furnace and your pituitary gland as the thermostat. Thyroid hormones are like heat: When the heat gets back to the thermostat, it turns the thermostat off and as the room cools (the thyroid hormone levels drop), the thermostat turns back on (TSH increases) and the furnace produces more heat (thyroid hormones).

The standard form of diagnosis is the thyroid-stimulating hormone or TSH test. This blood test measures how much TSH the pituitary is releasing, signaling the thyroid to release more T4. When an exhausted or defective thyroid doesn't respond to the pituitary's request for more T4, a biological "busy signal," so to speak, the pituitary releases more TSH. If its demands are still being ignored by the thy-

**TSH Normal Ranges**
*According to new guidelines issued in 2003, the normal TSH range is now 0.3 to 3.0 m/IU/L. This is lower than previous measurements.*

roid, the pituitary continues this pattern. High blood levels of TSH indicate a "no one home" signal from the thyroid, which is one indicator of hypothyroidism.

Normal ranges for TSH have recently been changed under the direction of the National Academy of Clinical Biochemistry, although many doctors are unaware of the changes that would place many more people in the range of low thyroid function. The new guidelines place the normal range at 0.3 to 3.0 m/IU/L. Anything higher than this can indicate hypothyroidism. This is also the target range for anyone on thyroid replacement.

The previous "normal" TSH ranges were 0.5 to 5.5 and endocrinologists now recommend a narrower range as indicative of hypothyroidism, and some even recommend lowering the upper limit to 2.5. This, Shomon says, would bring millions more people into the range of hypothyroidism and qualify them for treatment. If your doctor is unaware of the new guidelines, you can get a copy at www.nacb.org/lmpg/thyroid_LMPG_PDF.stm.

If your doctor tells you your TSH levels are "borderline" and refuses to treat you despite your symptoms, become proactive. Ask to know your actual numbers and ask for the "normal" ranges at the lab that did the testing. "If your doctor is so number obsessed that it's like talking to an accountant instead of a healthcare practitioner, start looking for a new doctor," advises Shomon.

You and your doctor should also be aware that TSH is not the only indicator of hypothyroidism. Many people with severe hypothyroidism can test within normal ranges for a variety of reasons, including the presence of a particularly insidious type of autoimmune thyroid disease called Hashimoto's (as previously mentioned). (You can learn more about Hashimoto's thyroiditis, Graves' disease, and hyperthyroidism—high thyroid function—in Chapter 6.)

## Testing T3 and T4

While the TSH is not the only test that can help diagnose hypothyroidism, your doctor may argue with you about this, too. Some doctors will be willing to measure T4 on the theory that low T4 levels and low test results on Free T4 are indicators of hypothyroidism.

However, like the TSH results, T4 levels can appear normal even when there is a severe deficiency. Measuring Total T3 or Free T3 is controversial and your doctor will likely tell you that these tests are not part of any conventional medical guidelines. Nevertheless, knowing these levels can be helpful in getting a diagnosis and may be helpful in diagnosing borderline cases.

**Free T3 and Free T4 Levels**

*The only accurate measure of active thyroid hormone levels in the blood. Free hormone levels tests frequently show abnormal free T3 and free T4 hormone levels below normal when TSH is in the normal range.*

Here are some ranges cited in my previous book, *8 Weeks to Vibrant Health*, written with Dr. Hyla Cass, that you should consider when your test results come back:

- T4 (total thyroxine): normal range is approximately 4.5–12.0 ug/dL. A reading of less than 4.5, along with high TSH, may indicate hypothyroidism. A low T4 with low TSH, may indicate a pituitary problem.

- Free T4: normal range is 0.7 to 1.53 ng/dL. Less than 0.7 may indicate hypothyroidism.

- Total T3 (total triiodothyronine): normal range is approximately 60–181 ng/dL. Less than 60 may indicate hypothyroidism. Optimal range is 120–124.

- Free T3: normal range is approximately 260–280 pg/mL. Less than 260 may indicate hypothyroidism.

- Reverse T3: this is a "false" T3 that the body produces during times of chronic stress or starvation (or overdieting). It takes up space on the T3 receptors, blocking the real T3 and preventing energy production. It's like applying the brakes in order to decrease energy expenditure.

- Anti-thyroid antibodies: will be elevated in autoimmune thyroiditis. Normal ranges are variable depending on the lab and on many other factors. For many people, elevated thyroid antibodies may be the only clue to their condition.

## Optimal Levels Are Individual

Each laboratory has a range of "normal" values and there is often a wide variance in ranges between labs. Some will tell you that a TSH result below 1.0 indicates hyperthyroid activity, while others say normal ranges can dip as low as 0.3.

Each individual is unique and laboratory values are far less important than what works for you. Some types of medications and supplements work wonderfully for some people, while other types of treatment work much better for others. Your doctor should consider your uniqueness and be willing to experiment with treatment options to determine what works best for you, not what a drug company representative is pushing this week.

## Home Tests

Thyroid hormone levels are usually tested by taking a blood sample, although saliva, urine, thermograph, and electro-acupuncture tests are also available. However, blood tests are the most commonly used and are generally considered to be reliable.

Thyroid function saliva tests are available and some natural practitioners think they are more accurate than blood tests. It will be a challenge to find a mainstream physician who uses them. However there are home test kits available that instruct you to make a simple finger stick to get a blood spot that can be used to analyze thyroid hormone levels.

Test kits can be obtained from companies like BioSafe's TSH test kit available at: http://www.test symptomsathome.com/BIO07.asp and ZRT's full panel thyroid hormone test that analyzes TSH, T4, T3, and antibodies, available at: www.bloodspot test.com.

## The Diet Test

Even with this battery of tests, you may be unable to get a diagnosis. As Drs. Richard and Karilee Shames say in *Thyroid Power,* "The greatest test of all is how you feel—and not a laboratory number." This does not mean that your doctor will give you thyroid hormone replacement therapy just because you have symptoms. Most won't, although there are a few who are willing to give you a few months on thyroid hormones to determine if they make you feel better.

Dr. Sanford Siegel, author of *Is Your Thyroid Making You Fat?*, suggests a twenty-eight-day test diet. It's a rigorous 1,000-calorie high-protein, low-carb diet that Siegel guarantees will cause you to lose weight. "If you have any degree of hypothyroidism, the weight loss will be less than expected. Indeed, that is why you will suspect hypothyroidism; it is because the weight loss is inadequate. No matter how meager, you will lose something on a diet of 1,000 calories a day. No one has a metabolism that low."

Siegel and many other doctors will prescribe thyroid-replacement hormones based on the twenty-eight-day diet test.

If you truly stick to the diet, you will get a powerful indication whether hypothyroidism is an underlying cause of your inability to lose weight. However, if excess weight isn't your problem, a 1,000-calorie diet will do little more than cause you to lose weight you don't need to lose; it will likely have little or no effect on your thyroid hormone production.

## What's Next?

Now that you're armed with a battery of test results,

what do you do with them? You've won at least a partial victory by getting your doctor to order the tests. Depending on the results, you may be home free and have a prescription in your hand for some sort of thyroid-replacement medication that should help you feel better soon. (More about prescription medicines in Chapter 7.)

But what if your results are "inconclusive," your doctor thinks a TSH of 2.0 is good enough, or your results do not show hypothyroidism, although you have several symptoms? It's essential for you to become proactive at this point. If you get a call from your doctor's office saying your thyroid tests came back "normal," ask for a copy of your test results. It's important to know the numbers and the values your particular lab uses to determine what is "normal" and what is not.

## Kinesiology

Many practitioners, including some conventionally trained doctors, use applied kinesiology as a diagnostic tool. Kinesiology, or muscle testing, is a means of evaluating normal and abnormal body function by testing the strength of muscle response to pressure applied by the practitioner, usually by attempting to move a rigidly extended arm.

Developed in 1964 by a Detroit chiropractor, Dr. George Goodheart, the principle has broadened to include evaluation of the nervous, vascular, and lymphatic systems, cerebrospinal fluid function, nutrition, and the effectiveness of acupuncture. Using the energetic resources of your body, an experienced practitioner can use this technique in addition to other lab tests, to determine what is happening in your body, what additional tests might help you as an individual, and what treatments may be valuable.

## How Do You Feel?

The real benchmark should be how you feel and whether a trial course of thyroid hormones gives you relief from your symptoms. Anything less is simply not acceptable.

Do you have a good relationship with your doctor? Do you feel you get all your doctor's time and attention during office visits? Are your doctor and office staff attentive, respectful, responsive, and helpful? Is your doctor willing to look at information you have gleaned from books and/or online? If you answered "no" to any of these questions, it's time to look for a new doctor.

If your doctor is rigid about new ideas, unwilling to consider your research, dismissive of your symptoms as "aging" or "depression" or "female problems," or is interested only in touting a certain medication, it's also time to look for a new doctor.

As I mentioned at the beginning of this chapter, documenting your doctor's refusal to treat for thyroid disease is a powerful way to win your case. Write letters, have them signed and dated and included in your chart. Keep signed copies for your records. You may need to use this as leverage to get your insurer to approve treatment or to approve a referral to another doctor.

If you have a choice, move on. You have a legal right to copies of your medical records. Request a copy and start looking. Your doctor's office may be permitted to charge a reasonable fee for copying records, but it will be worth it if you get the treatment you need.

## The Right Doctor

See the Resources section at the back of this book for information on finding the best doctors.

"A great doctor is one who is your partner, treats you with courtesy and respect, listens to you and incorporates you into the decision-making process," writes Shomon in *Living Well with Hypothyroidism*. Most importantly, says Dr. Teitelbaum, a good doctor will treat the patient's symptoms, not lab tests. If a treatment works, then it is the correct treatment for the problem.

## Elizabeth's Story

Depression can have a number of underlying causes, and hypothyroidism can be one that is often overlooked.

Elizabeth C. was in her mid-thirties when overwhelming depression struck suddenly. "I went to the max three times. I was truly ready to commit suicide," she recalls twenty years later. Conventional medicine had little to offer Elizabeth other than antidepressant drugs that were completely ineffective for her. She had three series of thyroid tests and doctors told her all of them were within "normal" ranges, so they were sure her thyroid wasn't the problem.

She had some other symptoms that kept this determined young journalist doggedly on her quest for a diagnosis. "I didn't sweat at all. Never. And that's really strange because I live in a very hot climate," she recalls.

At one point, she had even been diagnosed with lupus, happily a misdiagnosis, as it turned out.

Finally her quest led Elizabeth to a doctor who could help. She recalls dragging herself into his office twenty years ago. "I was 35, but I felt 95. I had absolutely no energy," she says. This doctor looked at her test results and decided to try a moderate dose of thyroid hormone. It worked like magic! "Within 20 minutes of the time I took the first pill, I started to sweat. You can't imagine how exciting that was for me," she says. Everything was rosy for Elizabeth from then on. A month later, she was back in her doctor's office with a bounce in her step: "I felt 35 again. In one month, I had shed the weight of 60 years." Not only had she regained her energy, Elizabeth had regained her life. The depression lifted within that first month and the gloom never descended again.

Now Elizabeth leads an active and healthy life. She takes one little thyroid pill a day and never looks back on those dark days before she learned what was shattering her life.

# CHAPTER 4

# WHO'S AT RISK?

**M**edical science has identified several factors that affect thyroid function and others that increase the risk of thyroid disease. The reasons for some of these proclivities for impaired thyroid function are unknown, but the patterns are clear. Basically, your biggest risks of developing thyroid disease result from your sex (higher risk for women), the presence of thyroid disease in your immediate family, and your exposure to toxic substances throughout your life.

Many experts, including Drs. Richard and Karilee Shames, authors of *Feeling Fat, Fuzzy or Frazzled?*, think our toxic world poses the greatest risk of thyroid disease. "One main cause of hypothyroidism is the increasing number of hormonally active substances in terms of synthetic chemicals polluting our air, food, and water," says Dr. Richard Shames. Shames says that PCBs (polychlorinated biphenyls) are particularly challenging for people who are prone to hypothyroidism. These toxins were used in hundreds of industrial and commercial applications including electrical, heat transfer, and hydraulic equipment; as plasticizers in paints, plastics, and rubber products; in pigments, dyes, and carbonless copy paper and many other applications. More than 1.5 billion pounds of PCBs were manufactured in the United States prior to the 1977 ban on its production.

**Polychlorinated Biphenyls (PCBs)**
*Environmentally harmful industrial chemicals that have persisted in the environment and in living tissues and that are found especially in aquatic systems.*

The Environmental Protection Agency says PCBs can cause a variety of health problems. Based on animal studies, PCBs have been shown to affect the immune, reproductive, nervous, and endocrine systems. Human studies support PCBs' potential to cause cancer and other devastating health problems. Sadly, if you were alive before 1977, you were most likely exposed to PCBs in household products that were found in virtually every home. Dr. Shames explains that PCBs and other toxins found in our environment can trigger the body's autoimmune response, causing, among other problems, hypothyroidism.

## Risk Factor Checklist

You have a higher risk of developing thyroid disease if:

- You have a family member with a thyroid problem.

- You have another pituitary or endocrine disease (that is, diabetes, celiac disease, or gluten intolerance, Addison's or Cushing's disease, polycystic ovary syndrome, chronic fatigue, fibromyalgia, and others).

- Your thyroid has been monitored in the past or you've been treated for any type of thyroid irregularities including hypo- or hyper-thyroidism, goiter, thyroid nodules, Hashimoto's disease, Graves' disease, postpartum depression, or elevated thyroid antibodies.

- You've had all or part of your thyroid removed because of a goiter or nodules.

- You've had all or part of your thyroid removed because of cancer.

- You've been treated with radioactive iodine for Graves' disease, hyperthyroidism, or cancer.

- You've been treated with antithyroid drugs like Tapazole or TPU for Graves' disease or hyperthyroidism.

- You've had a pituitary tumor and/or pituitary disease.

- You currently have a goiter or nodules.

- You or a family member have another auto-immune disease (such as rheumatoid arthritis or lupus).

- You've been diagnosed with chronic fatigue syndrome.

- You've been diagnosed with fibromyalgia.

- You're female.

- You're over sixty.

- You've recently had a baby.

- You're near menopause or are postmenopausal.

- You're a smoker or you've recently quit smoking.

- You've been exposed to radiation.

- You've been treated with lithium.

- You've been treated with a wide variety of drugs listed in Shomon's book, *Living Well with Hypothyroidism.*

- You've been exposed to certain chemicals (i.e., perchlorate or fluoride) by living in an area where soil or ground water is contaminated with these toxins.

## More Risks

This broad list of risk enhancers for hypothyroidism goes even deeper. If you've used sea vegetables or iodine to self-treat for low thyroid function or if you've eliminated iodized salt from your diet, your risk may be greater.

If you live or have lived in the U.S. "Goiter Belt," including the St. Lawrence River Valley, the Appalachian Mountains, the Great Lakes basin westward through Minnesota, South and North Dakota, Montana, Wyoming, the Rockies, noncoastal Oregon, Washington and British Columbia and southern

**West Nile Virus**
*A newly emergent virus, found throughout the United States, which is transmitted by bites of infected mosquitoes. It causes no symptoms in 80 percent of people exposed, but it can cause flu-like symptoms in some and more serious symptoms in others, including paralysis.*

Canada; and even if your mother lived in the Goiter Belt when she was pregnant with you, your risk is increased.

If you drink water that comes from the Colorado River or you eat produce that is irrigated with water from the Colorado River or you live in a area that has been sprayed for West Nile virus, your risk is increased substantially

## More High-Risk Regions

Your risk is increased if you lived near a nuclear power plant or if you have lived in or have even visited the following areas at these times:

- In or near Chernobyl in the weeks after the nuclear accident on April 26, 1986, including Belarus, Russian Federation, Ukraine (with reduced risk to those who lived in or visited Poland, Austria, Denmark, Finland, Germany, Greece, or Italy)

- Near or downwind from the former nuclear weapons plant at Hanford in southcentral Washington State in the 1940s through the 1960s, particularly from 1955 to 1965

- Near the Nevada nuclear test site in the 1950s and 1960s. Particularly high risk to those who lived in certain counties of Utah, Idaho, Montana, Colorado, and Missouri, east and north of the site.

## Risks Become Overwhelming

Even such seemingly unconnected factors as drinking alcohol during pregnancy or having a mother who drank alcohol when she was pregnant with you increases your risk of thyroid dysfunction.

If you grew up drinking flouridated water or using fluoridated toothpaste or had regular exposure to chlorine in swimming pools, or you have mercury amalgam fillings in your teeth, your risk is increased.

If you eat a lot of fish, broccoli, cauliflower, cabbage, millet, corn, carrots, soy products, peaches, strawberries, walnuts, spinach, peanuts, and other foods that virtually every knowledgeable health practitioner highly recommends as important for optimal health, you're at increased risk.

## More Risk Factors

Other risk factors include recent fevers, diarrhea, skin rash, joint pain, and severe or life-threatening snake bite. Serious trauma to the neck, such as a broken neck or whiplash from a car accident, is also a risk factor. This list is fairly overwhelming, but Shomon has a much more detailed checklist of symptoms and risk factors in her book, *Living Well with Hypothyroidism*. This list can help you identify your personal risk factors and, along with your extensive list of symptoms, this can go a long way toward helping your doctor to diagnose your problem.

## Almost All of Us Are at Risk

If you've read this list carefully, you'll see that almost everyone who lives in the United States or has spent any significant amount of time here has at least a small risk, but if you have any of these risk factors, no matter how remote they seem to you, alert your doctor to them. If your doctor pooh-poohs them as old wives tales, run, don't walk for the nearest exit. Your doctor is poorly educated and won't give you the treatment you need. This is not cause for freaking out or great alarm. It's simply a heads-up and a warning that you need to take action.

When you add together the lengthy list of symptoms of hypothyroidism and the risk factors involved, you can see why some doctors think hypothyroidism may be the most underdiagnosed medical condition around.

# CHAPTER 5

# FLUCTUATING ADRENAL AND SEX HORMONES

Thyroid hormone dysfunction rarely is a stand-alone problem. Since the entire endocrine gland system is a complex web of interrelationships, when one goes out of balance, all the others are affected. In fact, in their book *Feeling Fat, Fuzzy or Frazzled?*, Drs. Richard and Karilee Shames have devised a system of determining which hormones are out of whack and how to deal with them. The Shameses say the thyroid, adrenals and sex glands (ovaries and testes) are a "solid foundation upon which the rest of our hormonal and metabolic health is built."

## The Three-Legged Stool

They compare the function of these three glands to a three-legged stool, sturdy when all three legs are of equal length, but rickety when a leg is too short or too long.

Adrenal dysfunction is a sad manifestation of the stresses of modern life. The Shameses call adrenal dysfunction "the frazzled or emotional challenge," compared to the physical challenges of thyroid dysfunction and the mental challenges of sex hormone imbalances. "Low thyroid and low adrenal often go hand in hand," adds endocrinologist Ron Hunninghake, M.D.

## Adrenal Dysfunction

The adrenals are two tiny grape-sized glands that sit atop the kidneys, producing a number of important hormones that control metabolism, fluid balance, heart rate and blood pressure. They also control our response to stressors—the well-known "fight or flight" syndrome in which adrenaline produces a rush of energy and strength, the "super-human" powers that allow a mother to lift a car crushing her child. The adrenals also produce cortisol, a steroid hormone, that has its good side and its bad side.

**Cortisol**
*The body's natural stress-fighting and anti-inflammatory hormone.*

First the benefits of cortisol: It maintains our ability to react to stress and illness, process sugars, and keep blood pressure steady; to fight inflammation, have strong immune function, and distribute fat in the body.

The core of the adrenal gland produces adrenaline (sometimes called epinephrine). The outer part of the adrenal gland, the cortex, makes:

- Cortisol, the stress hormone

- DHEA, an energizing hormone that declines with age, hence the decline in energy with age

- Aldosterone, the hormone that maintains salt and water balance in your body

- Estrogen and testosterone, the primary sex hormones, in small amounts

## Cortisol, the Stress Hormone

We all have difficult lives these days. Emotional stress seems to be a "given" in most of our lives, considering the pressures of home life, relationships, and jobs. Most of us are quite familiar with this type of stress, but we may not realize that there are other stressors that take a toll on our health, too, including the physical challenges presented by environmental toxins and intense exercise, and even the physiological challenges of dieting or illness. Our bodies are designed to return to normal after stress, but when we pile stressor upon stressor, cortisol levels stay high, eventually leading to adrenal fatigue.

Holistic practitioners believe millions of Americans suffer from adrenal fatigue, but most conventional doctors won't treat the condition until the adrenal glands are in full collapse, a condition called Addison's disease.

## Symptoms of Adrenal Fatigue

Adrenal fatigue is a reality in our overstressed society when simple stress crosses the line and begins to affect these sensitive glands. If your energy lags during the day, you feel emotionally shaky, you sleep less than seven hours a night or your sleep quality is poor, you use caffeine or carbohydrates as energy boosters, or you can't lose weight no matter how much you diet, these are the primary indicators you have adrenal dysfunction.

Here are general symptoms of adrenal fatigue:

- Unexplained fatigue
- Difficulty getting up in the morning, even after a sufficient amount of sleep
- A feeling of being overwhelmed
- General feeling of being rundown
- Difficulty bouncing back from illness
- Repeated infections
- Inability to let stressors go
- Craving for salty and sweet high carbohydrate snacks
- Energy pickup after six p.m.
- General achiness
- Low blood sugar
- Low blood pressure
- Dizziness upon standing up suddenly
- Waking up in the early morning hours with anxiety

## Testing for Adrenal Dysfunction

You may have as much difficulty getting a doctor to

test your adrenal function as getting a true thyroid function panel, but even recalcitrant doctors may be surprised to find that the vast majority of their patients will test outside the normal ranges. In fact, Marcy Holmes, a women's health nurse practitioner and a certified menopause clinician at the Women to Women Clinic in Yarmouth, Maine, writes that tests show 99 percent of the women at her clinic have impaired adrenal function. What a commentary on the stressors of the modern world!

Conventional medicine places "normal" cortisol levels across a very broad range, but conventional doctors seldom track the adrenals' day-night pattern (called diurnal rhythm). In order to get accurate readings, cortisol levels must be tested at several times during the day and night. Cortisol levels are normally high in the morning to help you get going. They will be lower, but steady during the day to sustain your energy levels and then drop in the evening to help you get a restful night's sleep.

High daytime cortisol levels that rise at night are indicative of an early stage of adrenal stress, also

**Hyperadrenia**
*The medical*
*term for overactive*
*adrenal glands.*

known as hyperadrenia. In the middle stages of the disease, cortisol rises and falls unevenly, the body striving to balance. At this stage, many sufferers turn to caffeine and carbohydrates in an instinctive effort to boost their energy. This challenges the adrenals even more.

## Getting Treatment

Conventional doctors usually refuse to treat impaired adrenal function until a patient has reached the extreme point, sometimes called adrenal exhaustion or Cushing's disease or Addison's disease. Holistic practitioners contend that by treating adrenal stress in early stages, the condition can be reversed before it reaches crisis level.

Standard medical treatment for severe adrenal insufficiency involves replacing cortisol orally with hydrocortisone, a synthetic glucocorticoid, and aldosterone, if it is considered necessary.

### Saliva Testing of DHEA and Cortisol Levels

Saliva testing of DHEA and cortisol levels can help determine if you are suffering from toxic stress. Normal ranges follow.

**DHEA:**
Women ages 19–30: 29–781 mcg/dL
Women ages 31–50: 12–379 mcg/dL
Postmenopausal women: 30–260 mcg/dL

**Cortisol:**
Morning: 4.3–22.4 mcg/dL
Night: 3.1–16.7 mcg/dL

Another helpful test is the ACTH or adrenocorticotropic hormone measurement. In the test, a synthetic form of the pituitary signaller, ACTH, is injected and then blood and urine measurements of cortisol are taken. People with adrenal insufficiency will excrete little or no cortisol.

However, these "normal" ranges for any kind of hormone test can be deceptive, say Drs. Shames in *Feeling Fat, Fuzzy, or Frazzled?*: "With the current 'normal' ranges for hormone blood tests, the

---

**Self-Test for Adrenal Fatigue**

You'll need a blood pressure cuff and a helper to do this simple test.

- Lie on your back for at least five minutes. Have your helper record your blood pressure.

- Sit up quickly and have your blood pressure taken again.

- Stand up quickly and take it again.

In people without adrenal dysfunction, the blood pressure will rise between 4 and 10 points with each step. If your blood pressure drops for either or both of the last two measurements, it's a strong sign you have adrenal fatigue.

assumption seems to be that every person has the same genetic potential, inherited possibility, and life experience. In reality, nothing could be further from the truth."

Long-term elevated cortisol levels and adrenal fatigue can lead to serious health problems, including depression, alcoholism, substance abuse, anorexia nervosa, heavy smoking, cancer, ulcers, diabetes, chronic pain, strokes, cardiovascular accidents, Parkinson's, multiple sclerosis, skin conditions (psoriasis, acne, eczema), Alzheimer's, and AIDS.

## Treating Adrenal Fatigue Naturally

There are natural ways to treat adrenal fatigue. I won't go into them in detail here, but you can research them for yourself. Some of the most commonly used supplements to promote adrenal health are dessicated adrenal glandular (sold over the counter, as are the thyroid glandulars described in Chapter 8), holy basil, rhodiola, ashwagandha, schizandra, wild oats, phosphorylated serines, low-dose compounded DHEA, cordyceps, bacopa, Siberian ginseng, glycerated licorice (full strength licorice extract) and pregnenolone.

The Shameses like to give their patients extra vitamin $B_5$ (pantothenic acid) and $B_6$ (pyridoxine) and they recommend a product called SeriPhos, phosphylated brand of the nutritional amino acid serine, one of the few over-the counter remedies for excessive cortisol. They recommend taking 1,000 milligrams an hour before the time your test results showed the highest cortisol readings.

You can also get a high quality adrenal glandular called IsoCort by prescription or liquid adrenal glandulars sold by prescription in compounding pharmacies.

Dr. Teitelbaum recommends 2 to 3 grams of licorice root twice a day for not more than six to eight weeks, adding 100 milligrams of Asian ginseng after four to six weeks, 325 to 650 milligrams of echinacea three times daily and 500 to 2,000 milligrams of vitamin C daily. For more details on this plan, see Dr. Teitelbaum's book, *From Fatigued to Fantastic.*

## Dietary Recommendations

Many practitioners recommend eliminating coffee and artificial sweeteners, adding a high potency multivitamin, consuming a low carbohydrate diet, engaging in stress management techniques, increasing exercise, and getting more sleep if you have adrenal insufficiency.

The Shameses also suggest eating six small meals a day rather than three larger ones and, if your blood pressure is under 135/85, to consider *adding* salt to your diet—but use sea salt without iodine added. The small amount of iodine naturally found in sea salt is not a problem.

## Menopause and More

Since we already know that women are far more susceptible to thyroid dysfunction than men, and perimenopausal and postmenopausal women have an even higher risk, it stands to reason that there is a connection between these thyroid and sex hormones. Although medical science hasn't yet pinpointed the precise point of interaction, the link is fairly well established in scientific literature. Here's what we do know: Estrogen suppresses thyroid function and progesterone enhances or stabilizes it.

Some practitioners think the thyroid may actually be working properly during perimenopause, but excess free estrogen that usually accompanies menopause is blocking the thyroid hormones from working effectively, a thyroid hormone resistance similar to insulin resistance that develops into type 2 diabetes.

In his book, *Solving the Riddle of Illness,* Dr. Stephen Langer says, "Distinguishing the influences of menopause from those of hypothyroidism relative to symptoms of middle-aged women is not unlike trying to perform surgery to part Siamese twins—it is extremely difficult."

## Sex-Hormone Replacement Is Not Enough

In 1999, the American Association of Clinical Endocrinologists (AACE) alerted its members that hormone replacement alone is frequently not enough to manage the symptoms of menopause and menopause-like symptoms. The AACE advised its member doctors that such women may be suffering from undiagnosed hypothyroidism. Remember we noted the symptoms of hypothyroidism and perimenopause have great similarities? The AACE currently recommends that perimenopausal women add thyroid hormone replacement to the list of hormones they discuss with their doctors.

Seven years ago, endocrinologists were advised to warn their patients of this possibility—yet how many do? In fact, how many perimenopausal women get to see an endocrinologist for their symptoms? Precious few. The word needs to get out far beyond the 4,000 doctors who are part of the AACE. It needs to be in the hands of the tens of thousands of primary care doctors, gynecologists, internal medicine specialists and all healthcare professionals who treat perimenopausal and postmenopausal women. And most important, the information needs to be in the hands of the women who need this help.

## Perils of Perimenopause

Here's a simple explanation of what's happening during perimenopause. The time period preceding menopause is not a simple matter of nosediving estrogen production. One of the first clinical signs of menopause is a gradual decline in progesterone levels. At the same time, estrogen levels may remain stable or even increase slightly. To further complicate matters, estrogen is actually a group of several hormones, any one of which can become unbalanced. Progesterone and estrogen play a delicate balancing act throughout the menstrual cycle, rising and falling as the cycle progresses. Without sufficient progesterone, estrogen becomes dominant.

Here's an explanation of what Marla Ahlgrimm calls "the estrogen/progesterone *pas de deux*" in her book, *The HRT Solution*. First, estrogen causes an increase in endometrial cell production; progesterone protects the endometrium from this kind of cell growth. Second, estrogen can suppress the action of your thyroid gland, while progesterone can enhance it. Finally, estrogen increases salt and fluid retention; progesterone, on the other hand, works like a diuretic, prompting the body to excrete fluids. The uncomfortable symptoms of peri-menopause are actually the result of excess estrogen, so, for most women, estrogen-based hormone replacement alone isn't helpful at all.

As a woman moves further into perimenopause, progesterone continues its decline while estrogen levels begin to swing like a pendulum, and instead of releasing one mature egg, the ovaries begin to release whole groups of mature eggs each month.

At the same time, we begin to see seesawing levels of FSH (follicular-stimulating hormone) and LH (luteinizing hormone), the hormones that are normally released by the pituitary gland to help the egg mature and to regulate ovulation.

## Synthetic Hormone Replacement

Most of us know that the standard medical treatment of symptoms of perimenopause is still synthetic hormone replacement, most often from the urine of pregnant mares. These types of hormones have been largely discredited in recent years when studies showed they actually increased the risk of heart attacks, strokes, cancer, and Alzheimer's disease, despite decades of medical promises that they protect against these dread diseases.

Fortunately, there are many safe and effective natural alternatives for perimenopausal and menopausal symptoms. Among them are black cohosh, red clover, vitex (chasteberry), soy isoflavones, coenzyme $Q_{10}$, L-carnitine, dong quai, DHEA, evening primrose oil, and many more.

There are also natural forms of prescription hormone replacement, also known as bioidentical hormones, available through compounding pharmacies. They are made from a soy base altered to precisely mimic the hormones of a thirty-five-year-old woman. They are regulated by the FDA and are only available by prescription.

For more information, see my book, *User's Guide to Natural Hormone Replacement*.

## Catch-22

Here's the kicker: When your thyroid isn't functioning well, it challenges your adrenals, and, conversely, when your adrenals are fatigued or overstressed, thyroid function is threatened. Remember Richard and Karilee Shameses' three-legged stool? You've got a really rickety platform for the energy system of your body if you have low thyroid and elevated cortisol stressing your adrenals. And we already know that adrenal fatigue adversely affects thyroid function, so these two glandular functions definitely go hand in hand. Treating thyroid and not adrenals can overstimulate the already overworked adrenals, creating even more imbalance in your system. Add to that the fact that perimenopausal and menopausal women are at high risk for depressed thyroid function and you can see there is a strong connection between thyroid and sex hormones, making that three-legged stool even more shaky.

The Shameses say: "While we can't see emotions or the biochemicals that cause them, we know they exist, and we can see their effects on our behaviors. Similarly while we cannot see the hormones flowing in our bloodstream, we can see their 'footprints' in certain health patterns."

Doctors are not trained to consider the three energy hormones and the delicate balance that they must achieve in order to keep your energy at optimum levels. Since your doctor is unlikely to suggest a full hormone panel, including thyroid, adrenal, and sex hormones, it's up to you to push for it. The results of these tests will give you some insight into your health challenges, but remember, many people have impaired hormonal function even if it doesn't appear on tests. Your best option is to find a doctor who will prescribe the hormones you need on a trial basis, see if you feel better and be willing to make adjustments until you find out what works.

## Chronic Fatigue and Fibromyalgia

Chronic fatigue syndrome and fibromyalgia are two conditions with similar symptoms which have many symptoms in common with hypothyroidism. Dr. Teitelbaum names "the autoimmune triad," a set of conditions that triggers an autoimmune response to thyroid and adrenal glands and in the body cells that assist in the absorption of vitamin $B_{12}$. That's why, says Dr. Teitelbaum, so many chronic fatigue and fibromyalgia patients have thyroid and adrenal problems. "When the body attacks these 'invaders,' the resulting low levels of thyroid and adrenal hormones and vitamin $B_{12}$ trigger fibromyalgia and poor sleep, which then suppresses the hypothalamus gland, setting the fatigue cycle in motion," he says in *From Fatigued to Fantastic.*

There's a sex hormone component to the chronic fatigue/fibromyalgia syndrome, says Dr. Teitelbaum, that comes from low estrogen levels that can occur ten to fifteen years before "official" menopause.

Dr. Stephen Langer closely links the deep muscle, bone, and even tendon pain of fibromyalgia with hypothyroidism. In his practice, Dr. Langer says, he frequently recommends the Barnes Basal Body Temperature Test (see page 24) to people who complain of this type of pain and of crushing fatigue—and the majority of time, he finds they have low body temperatures, a positive indicator for hypothyroidism. Three of four fibromyalgia patients Dr. Langer treats with Armour thyroid have responded well, he writes in *Solved: The Riddle of Illness.*

He cites a study by Dr. John Lowe, director of research for the Fibromyalgia Research Foundation, that offers a suggestion that fibromyalgia is actually untreated hypothyroidism that causes a deficiency of thyroid hormones and cellular resistance to thyroid hormones. Dr. Lowe found that 63 percent of the thirty-eight fibromyalgia patients he studied were deficient in thyroid hormones. Their symptoms included poor sleep, fatigue, aches and pains, cold sensitivity, depression, and brain fog. Sound familiar? There's certainly a pattern here.

Among the natural approaches to chronic fatigue and fibromyalgia are NADH (nicotinamide adenine dinucleotide), creatine, coenzyme $Q_{10}$, ginger, gingko, kava kava, tyrosine, valerian, and lemon balm.

# CHAPTER 6

# OTHER TYPES OF THYROID DYSFUNCTION

While hypothyroidism is by far the most common form of thyroid dysfunction, there are some others you should know about.

## Hashimoto's Thyroiditis

Hashimoto's is a form of hypothyroidism caused by autoimmune system malfunction. You probably remember that some experts say all or almost all forms of hypothyroidism have an autoimmune component, but Mary Shomon, herself a sufferer of Hashimoto's, explains the difference. "Hashimoto's and hypothyroidism are not interchangeable terms. Hashimoto's is a disease. Hypothyroidism is a condition. Hashimoto's is an autoimmune disease that *usually* causes people to eventually become hypothyroid. Hypothyroidism is a condition that can result from a number of causes and diseases."

This form of hypothyroidism is an inherited form of autoimmune disease that results in an impairment of the thyroid-hormone producing cells, say the Shameses in *Feeling Fat, Fuzzy or Frazzled?* People with Hashimoto's have reduced amounts of T3 and T4, resulting in the classic symptoms of hypothyroidism, especially difficulty regulating temperature and experiencing low energy.

Sometimes, as the thyroid is in the process of failing, it will kick into overdrive, causing symptoms of hyperthyroidism, a difficult to diagnose condition known as hashitoxicosis.

However, eventually Hashimoto's disease burns out the thyroid gland, leaving it functioning at a very low level or not at all.

### Hashimoto's Symptoms

Some people with Hashimoto's report that they feel exhausted, yet "stuck in high gear." That's because Hashimoto's has elements of hyperthyroidism and hypothyroidism at the same time, say the Shameses in *Thyroid Power*. "It is as if a car is stuck in neutral, with the engine racing, but no movement. Some describe feeling as if there is one foot on the brake and the other on the gas," they wrote.

Goiter or an enlargement of the thyroid gland is often present in people with Hashimoto's. Thyroiditis attacks can occur when the thyroid becomes severely inflamed. Dr. Stephen Langer, author of *Solved: The Riddle of Illness*, refers to thyroiditis as "arthritis of the thyroid." He says thyroiditis can mean pain and inflammation in the thyroid for some sufferers just like arthritis means pain and inflammation in the joints. During a thyroiditis attack, common symptoms are similar to those of hyperthyroidism: anxiety, panic attacks, heart palpitations, swelling in the thyroid area, problems swallowing, and frequently, disrupted sleep patterns.

Managing Hashimoto's may mean treating both high and low thyroid, but it's essential to arrive at a solid diagnosis of Hashimoto's before and ruling out some of the hyperthyroid conditions mentioned in the following pages before any irreversible treatment, such as radiation, is considered. (See discussion about radiation treatment later in this chapter.)

### Diagnosis

Autoimmune thyroid disease is diagnosed through thyroid-antibody testing. People with this condition will often have TSH levels within normal ranges. Thyroid antibodies, coupled with symptoms of hypothyroidism, signal that the thyroid is failing due to an autoimmune response. The body has, for some inexplicable reason, decided the thyroid is a foreign invader that must be vanquished. Some doctors will order additional tests to confirm a diagnosis of Hashimoto's, including thyroglobulin and thyroid peroxidase antibodies, antithyroglobulin, antithyrotropin receptor-blocking antibodies, anti-TSH antibody, and anti-T4 and anti-T-3 antibodies.

The simplest means of diagnosis is the presence of a goiter. Some doctors will do a fine needle aspiration of the thyroid, looking for the presence of lymphocytes and macrophages typical of Hashimoto's. Others prefer an ultrasound to confirm an enlarged thyroid or a radioactive scan that would show impaired uptake in the enlarged thyroid.

This battery of tests is likely to present a better picture of what's happening, if you are lucky enough to find a doctor who takes the time to prescribe them and read them.

### Risk Factors

The biggest risk for Hashimoto's is being female, since 75 percent of sufferers of all autoimmune diseases are women, most of them in their childbearing years. You're also at greater risk of Hashimoto's if you have a family history of any of the following autoimmune diseases: endometriosis, rheumatoid arthritis, multiple sclerosis, psoriasis, lupus, Sjögren's syndrome, Raynaud's disease, or vitiligo. Conversely, if you are diagnosed with Hashimoto's your risk of the above diseases increases.

Sadly, as you have no doubt already discovered if you've shuttled from doctor to doctor, getting a diagnosis and then getting appropriate treatment is not an easy matter. Many doctors are resistant to testing for thyroid antibodies if TSH levels are in the normal range. Some even believe that a positive test for thyroid antibodies is not enough to prescribe thyroid hormones. You may have to doctor shop in order to find a doctor willing to do the regular monitoring necessary with the hormone swings characteristic of Hashimoto's so you can be given the proper treatment.

### Treatment

Thyroid hormone replacement is necessary for anyone suffering from Hashimoto's. You'll learn more about types of treatment in Chapter 7. Some doctors use complementary therapies, like acupuncture, to stimulate TSH, and the use of proper diet and supplements can also be helpful, as you'll learn in Chapters 8 and 9.

## Hyperthyroidism

Hyperthyroidism is the direct opposite of hypothyroidism. It's an overactive thyroid that is producing too much thyroid hormone. It can speed up all body processes, including heart rate and blood pressure, sometimes to dangerous levels.

Graves' disease, an autoimmune condition also sometimes known as diffuse toxic goiter, is the most common type of hyperthyroidism. However, hyperthyroidism can also be caused by toxic nodules or goiters on the thyroid, excessive thyroid hormone replacement given to hypothyroidism suffers, iodine excess, and thyroiditis or an inflammation of the thyroid.

**Graves' Disease**
*A common form of hyperthyroidism, characterized by goiter and often a slight protrusion of the eyeballs; it is also called Basedow's disease and exophthalmic goiter.*

Graves' can be triggered by stress; smoking; radiation to the neck; some medications, including interleukin-2, commonly taken for immune deficiency diseases like HIV and some types of cancer; and interferon-alpha, used to treat certain types of cancer and hepatitis C and to prevent rejection of organ transplants.

### Symptoms

It would stand to reason that the symptoms of hyperthyroidism would be the complete opposite of those of hypothyroidism. Not true. In fact, some are remarkably similar.

Here are some of the most common symptoms of hyperthyroidism:

• nervousness

- irritability and restlessness
- fatigue
- increased perspiration and heat intolerance
- thinning of skin or velvety textured skin
- fine, brittle hair
- depression
- muscular weakness especially involving the upper arms and thighs
- shaky hands
- sweaty palms
- panic disorder
- insomnia
- racing heart
- more frequent bowel movements
- weight loss despite an increased appetite
- lighter menstrual flow, less frequent periods
- bulging or protruding eyes
- blurred vision
- red, inflamed eyes
- double vision
- rarely, a reddish, lumpy thickening of the skin on the shins

Like other thyroid disorders, hyperthyroidism is far more common in women than in men, with women bearing the brunt by 8:1. It typically occurs in middle age, again suggesting a link between thyroid hormone imbalance and female sex hormones that begin to fluctuate in middle age when perimenopause begins.

### Diagnosis

Unlike hypothyroidism, hyperthyroidism is usually easily diagnosed by a physical examination in which one or more of the following are present:

- enlarged thyroid gland
- rapid heart beat (tachycardia) or heart palpitations
- smooth, velvety skin
- tremor of the fingertips
- for Graves' disease, bulging eyes and skin problems as described above

Blood tests for TSH, T3 and T4 are fairly definitive diagnostic tools. An exceptionally low TSH is a certain indicator of hyperthyroidism.

### Treatment

Conventional medicine treats hyperthyroidism with a course of antithyroid drugs such as propylthiouracil (PTU) and methimazole (Tapazole). These drugs slow the thyroid's absorption of iodine, thus slowing thyroid hormone production. These drugs can cause a dramatically lowered white blood cell count and a skin rash.

Hyperthyroidism can be a very serious and even life-threatening condition, and ignoring the symptoms can be dangerous. However, in 25 percent of the cases, the symptoms disappear on their own, so doctors are increasingly giving hyperthyroidism the "wait and see" treatment. Treatment—or lack of it—needs to be very closely supervised by a doctor.

The most common conventional medical treatment for hyperthyroidism is radiation iodine (RAI) treatment that destroys the thyroid gland, leaving you hypothyroid and in need of thyroid hormone replacement medications for life, a drastic measure that should be considered very carefully before you take it. The radioactive pills are taken by mouth and the radioactive iodine goes from the stomach to the bloodstream and eventually into the thyroid gland. The RAI is attracted to the thyroid from the bloodstream for the production of thyroid hormone. Once it is in the thyroid, the radioactivity destroys thyroid cells, reducing and eventually stopping production of thyroid hormone. RAI is usually administered in a single dose and relief takes three to six months. Sometimes, if the dosage was too low, a second dose may be administered.

The problem with RAI is that it is difficult to control the rate at which thyroid cells are destroyed by the radioactive iodine, and this result eventually puts most people who started with hyperthyroidism in a hypothyroid state.

The final option for hyperthyroidism is surgery to remove part of the thyroid gland in an effort to control the overactivity. The amount to remove is somewhat arbitrarily arrived at and frequently people who opt for surgery instead of RAI will require thyroid hormone replacement for the rest of their lives.

### The Risks

Ignoring the symptoms or self-treating hyperthyroidism can be very dangerous. While you might start out with some uncomfortable symptoms like an irregular heart beat, untreated hyperthyroidism can lead to chest pain, high blood pressure, possible severe emotional disorders, heart failure, and even death.

When the thyroid becomes so seriously accelerated, it's called a thyroid crisis or thyroid storm, a medical emergency that requires urgent treatment.

Thyroid storm is not common—it only affects 1 to 2 percent of people with hyperthyroidism and is more common in the elderly. Mary Shomon says, "During a thyroid storm, the heart rate, blood pressure and body temperature can become uncontrollably high. Whenever thyroid storm is suspected, the patient must go immediately on an emergency basis to the hospital, as this is a life-threatening condition that can develop and

**Thyroid Storm**
*A sudden life-threatening exacerbation of the symptoms of hyperthyroidism, such as high fever, tachycardia, weakness, or extreme restlessness, that can be brought on by infection, surgery, or stress.*

worsen quickly and requires treatment within hours to avoid fatal complications such as stroke or heart attack."

The vast majority of people with hyperthyroidism never experience a crisis. Yet doctors often rush even mild cases to treatment, perhaps to the patient's disadvantage, says Elaine Moore, author of *Graves' Disease: A Practical Guide.*

"Even though it's been long known that a number of people with Graves' disease achieve spontaneous remission without treatment, some doctors think that hypothyroidism is preferable to hyperthyroidism. People like me who have mild symptoms are having their thyroid glands destroyed although wiser doctors monitor symptoms and determine the disease's natural progression before even suggesting treatment," she says.

### Natural Options

The German Commission E has described certain herbs as both safe and effective for the treatment of hyperthyroidism, yet few doctors in the United States are familiar with herbal therapy. "They object to trying something new although they don't think twice about destroying the thyroid of someone with subclinical or mild symptoms. The moderators of one popular thyroid board (online discussion) do a great disservice to Graves' disease patients in that they try to scare people into having aggressive treatment by suggesting that the rare condition of thyroid storm is a common event, and they refuse to publish reports of spontaneous remission," says Moore. She continues, "They ban reports, even published studies, listing the benefits of alternative medicine and pull posts of patients who object to the use of radioiodine. There are several support groups who receive funding from drug companies and consequently perpetuate the notion that hypothyroidism is a simple, easily treated condition."

Among the herbs that have been recommended to treat hyperthyroidism are bugleweed, motherwort, turmeric, milk thistle, hawthorn berry, lemon balm, and licorice. Quercetin, a bioflavonoid, found in apples, onions, and garlic, can also be very helpful.

Homeopathic remedies such as Calcarea phos, Calcarea carb, Lapis alb, Iodium, Thyroidinum, Spongia, Lycopus, and Calcarea iod may also be helpful.

Many patients have found relief from their symptoms with massage, acupuncture, and craniosacral therapy.

# CHAPTER 7

# CONVENTIONAL MEDICINE'S APPROACH TO HYPOTHYROIDISM

Conventional medicine, when it treats hypothy-roidism, prefers to treat it with synthetic thyroid hormones. The most common treatment is with levothyroxine, which is synthetic T4, and which is the generic name for brands like Synthroid, Levoxyl, Levothroid, Levothyroid, and Euthyrox.

Synthroid, which contains no T3, is a top-selling thyroid hormone in the United States. It is a little more expensive than the other T4 products, but otherwise differs little from them except in fillers and binders and the time they take to dissolve.

Consistency in dosage and potency was the subject of a prolonged battle between manufacturers of the levothyroxine drugs and the FDA. These drugs had been "grandfathered" into approval under the approval given a century ago to Armour thyroid. It's an interesting paradox that while drug companies have insisted that it is Armour thyroid that is dosage inconsistent, the FDA determined that the synthetics were inconsistent in dosage and forced them to go through the FDA approval process all over again a few years ago. After a great deal of argument, deadline extensions, FDA warnings, and general weeping and wailing and gnashing of teeth on the part of the drug companies, these synthetics were approved again, although there are still frequent recalls of these products due to potency and stability problems.

In her book, *Living Well with Hypothyroidism*, Mary Shomon says that while levothyroxine products have some variations in potency from batch to batch, brand names have fewer variations than

generic products. "Most doctors do not recommend or prescribe generic levothyroxine anyway,
but pharmacies often will substitute them. Some
health maintenance organizations insist on the
cheaper generic when a brand name has been prescribed. *Do not accept generic levothyroxine, if at
all possible,* and always be sure to check your prescription every time you get it filled to make sure
the pharmacy hasn't substituted generic for brand
name," Shomon writes. If your insurance company
gives you no other option, pay for your thyroid
medication yourself. It's cheap. Synthroid, the most
expensive is about $14 for a month's supply of a typ-
ical dose; Levoxyl is about $11. In addition, some
people are allergic to the fillers in some brands and
that problem can be relieved by switching to another brand.

## The Research Wars

Millions of prescriptions have been written for these
drugs because modern physicians have been educated to believe that this treatment offers the best
results, so a shock wave went through the medical
community in 1999 with the release of an important
study that showed that treating hypothyroidism
with T4 hormone alone was not nearly as effective
as treating it with a combination of T3 and T4.

Yet most doctors will still tell you that sufficient
synthetic T4 converts well to T3. The results of this
landmark study were met with resistance, and
according to Shomon, "Since anything that will take
away business from the levothyroxine manufacturers has got to be a threat, it's no surprise that after
the 1999 study was published, teams of researchers
set out to defend against the threat and prove that
levothyroxine should be the only game in town."

Three subsequent studies, published as part of
the research wars of 2003, showed that a combination of T3 and T4 was not superior to T4 alone.
Score one for the drug companies. Shomon says,
"Aside from the politics, there is a real question

about the validity and quality of the (2003) studies, and whether they prove anything about T3. Many of the experts who regularly prescribe T3 say the studies are seriously flawed and don't prove anything . . . Among those flaws, says Shomon, are the incorrect dosages of T3 used in the study; the variations of what is now considered the "normal ranges"; the "one size fits all" study approach that prevented patients from getting dosages that might be more helpful; a study size that is too small, a contradiction of clinical experience of thousands of doctors and clinicians; and the fact that the 1999 study was not the first to suggest that T3, in addition to T4, was necessary for optimal results for hypothyroid patients.

Dr. David Brownstein, author of *The Miracle of Natural Hormones*, says the real flaw of the 2003 studies was that the wrong type of T3 was used. He wrote, "I have not found that much benefit from adding T3. But I have found the desiccated thyroid much more effective. My clinical experience has shown that desiccated thyroid is very effective and clinically seems to have better response than using T4 therapy alone."

In addition, Dr. Shames notes, "It doesn't really matter what the research says. What works is all that matters. If it helps a patient feel better, that's what I will go with." In addition, according to Dr. Stephen Langer, nothing much is going to be helpful if there is untreated adrenal dysfunction that accompanies a large percentage of hypothyroidism.

---

### Take Them First Thing

It's best to take thyroid hormones on an empty stomach first thing in the morning. If you're taking any kind of thyroid hormones, be sure to take them at least three hours apart from multivitamins and minerals, since iron and calcium block the absorption of the hormones.

In his book, *Solved: The Riddle of Illness*, Dr. Langer says, "When the adrenal system is weak or exhausted even from the various physical, emotional or mental stresses—even the mildest adrenal insufficiency—it must be strengthened before or during thyroid treatment for the treatment to be effective."

## Desiccated Thyroid—the Natural Way

So what is this strange stuff?

Desiccated thyroid isn't strange or new at all. In fact, dessicated thyroid has been on the market for more than one hundred years, and one brand, Armour thyroid, was the only thyroid hormone replacement therapy available until 1950, when the synthetics came on the market.

Because it is natural, Armour thyroid probably should be included in the next chapter on natural therapies, but it's also a prescription drug for which 2 million prescriptions were written in 2003. That's a substantial number in the more-or-less conventional market, but a tiny drop in the bucket compared to 52 million prescriptions for Synthroid in the same time period. Made from pig thyroid glands, Armour thyroid, as a prescription drug, is regulated by the FDA and standardized for potency, despite what your doctor might believe, and what you might be told by those who have been unduly influenced by the manufacturers of synthetic thyroid hormones. Armour is still the most commonly prescribed natural thyroid hormone replacement drug on the market, but there are a handful of other desiccated thyroid preparations, including Naturethroid (hypoallergenic) and Westhroid. There is a generic "Thyroid Strong," a Parke-Davis natural desiccated thyroid product and another brand, Biotech. All of these pork-based thyroid medications contain T3 and T4 in standardized quantities.

Your doctor may tell you that the quantities of hormones in Armour thyroid fluctuate from batch to batch, but this is drug industry propaganda.

Armour thyroid meets stringent USP (United States Pharmacoepeia) standards, mixing different lots from different animals to achieve a consistent quality. There are also periodic rumors that Armour thyroid has been infected with bovine spongiform encephalopathy (BSE) or mad cow disease. This is patently absurd because Armour comes from the thyroid glands of pigs, not cows, and pigs have never been known to contract BSE. Your doctor may also tell you that desiccated thyroid may go off the market. This completely unfounded rumor appears to have been started by competing drug companies, says Mary Shomon.

## Synthetic T3 and T4

The majority of synthetic thyroid hormones on the market contain only T4, counting on the body to convert the T4 to T3. That will be effective if your body is converting hormones properly. When the conversion doesn't work properly, some holistic practitioners think T3 is the answer. There are two synthetic products on the market that provide T3 and a combination of T3 and T4. Liothyronine is a synthetic T3 marketed under the brand name Cytomel, and liotrix (Thyrolar) is a synthetic T3/T4. If your doctor is completely resistant to desiccated thyroid, you may be more successful in obtaining a prescription for the synthetic versions.

Cytomel and Thyrolar are most frequently prescribed by holistic practiioners. Hormones containing T3 are also sometimes used to treat persistent depression in people with hypothyroidism and sometimes even in those without hypothyroidism.

## Osteoporosis

Some doctors justify keeping TSH levels somewhat high because of studies that suggest that levothyroxine can increase the risk of osteoporosis. Thyroid hormone replacement will be needed after a person with hyperthyroidism develops hypothyroidism as a result of treatment, and extremely low TSH levels, which can be caused by swinging hormones as the thyroid fails, may increase the risk of osteoporosis.

Mary Shomon says, "While the research is contradictory, some doctors only hear the findings that show very low TSH levels increase osteoporosis risk. Based on limited information, these doctors then compound the problem by employing faulty logic: If a very low TSH level poses a risk, then why not keep people at *higher* levels and thereby avoid the risk (of osteoporosis)? Hence the current penchant to medicate patients only to high-normal TSH levels. These patients then walk around feeling unwell, being told it's not their thyroid, with the doctor refusing to prescribe a higher dose of thyroid hormone." However, later research and re-analysis of earlier research suggests there are no negative effects of levothyroxine on bone density. If you are concerned about osteoporosis or you are at risk for the disease, you can take 1,500 to 2,000 milligrams of highly absorbable calcium daily. Be sure to add at least 400 milligrams of magnesium and 400 IU of vitamin D to ensure the calcium will be absorbed.

**Osteoporosis**
*A condition that affects especially older women and is characterized by a decrease in bone mass with decreased bone density and enlargement of bone spaces producing porosity and fragility.*

# CHAPTER 8

# NATURAL THYROID REMEDIES

**A**s I mentioned in Chapter 7, Armour thyroid is certainly at the top of the list of prescription thyroid-replacement hormones that are natural, safe, and effective.

However, if you're not yet ready to go the prescription route, your thyroid dysfunction is marginal, or you can't get a doctor to confirm a diagnosis with a prescription for thyroid hormones, there are a relatively large number of supplements and herbs that have been shown to be helpful.

## High Quality Multivitamins

Before we start on the list, let me say you need a high-quality multivitamin if you're not already taking one. What does "high-quality" mean? Look for one that comes close to the following shopping list of essential nutrients. You may not find a single product that contains these precise amounts, but look for something that comes as close as possible.

Look for a product that is natural, simply because it will not contain artificial coloring, preservatives, sugar, starch, coal tar, and other additives you would prefer to avoid.

A day's dosage of a good multivitamin should contain:

- Vitamin A            5,000–10,000 IU

- Beta-carotene       10,000–25,000 IU

- Vitamin C            500–1,000 mg

- Vitamin D            400–800 IU

- Vitamin E            200–600 IU

- Thiamin                50–100 mg
- Riboflavin             50–100 mg
- Niacin                 50–100 mg
- Vitamin B$_6$          50–100 mg
- Folic acid             400–800 mcg
- Vitamin B$_{12}$       50–100 mg
- Biotin                 10–50 mcg
- Pantothenic acid       10–50 mg
- Inositol               10–25 mg
- PABA                   10–25 mg
- Calcium                1,500 mg
- Magnesium              250–500 mg
- Zinc                   15–50 mg
- Copper                 0.5–2 mg
- Manganese              5–15 mg
- Boron                  1–3 mg
- Selenium               50–200 mcg
- Iodine                 50–150 mcg
- Chromium               50–200 mcg

## What's Best for Hypothyroidism

If you have been diagnosed with hypothyroidism and/or if your symptoms suggest this is your problem, chose one or two of the herbs or supplements from the following list and see if you find relief. It's

---

**Unit Measures—International Units (IU), Milligrams (mg), and Micrograms (mcg)**

These units measure vitamins and minerals by potency or weight. All three are extremely small amounts (milligrams are one-thousandth of a gram; micrograms are one-millionth of a gram). For example 400 micrograms is about 1/70,000th of an ounce.

not a good idea to take large amounts of these or
to take a dozen different things at once. Try one or
two or try a carefully balanced combination like
Thyro-Sense. You may need to devise your own
trial-and-error method to determine what works
best for you.

### Treatments for Hypothyroidism

The following supplements can help relieve the
symptoms of hypothryoidism.

**Thyroid glandulars.** These are actual thyroid hormone tissues of animal origin with most of the
active ingredients removed so they can be sold
without a prescription. The Shameses say the extra
raw materials and building blocks provided by the
glandular substance often have a positive effect on
a sluggish thyroid system. There has been research
that suggests that even a tiny amount of assistance
with thyroid hormone levels can be enough to
reduce the autoimmune response the Shameses
think is behind most cases of hypothyroidism.

Elson Haas, M.D. author of *Staying Healthy with
Nutrition* (Celestial Arts, 1992), says these glandulars once seemed incredible to him, but he now has
more information: "On the positive side, it is likely
that the basic components of those gland tissues
may offer the precursor substances that our own
bodies and glands can use to enhance their functions. And there may be hidden factors that may
offer some benefit. The glands, like foods, supply
basic nutrients, such as amino acids, oils, vitamins,
other active ingredients and a potential 'life force,'
where a drug will not. Some evidence from radio-
isotope studies suggests that glands, when eaten,
do in fact get to the human glands and influence
them."

**L-Tyrosine.** This key amino acid helps the thyroid
gland manufacture sufficient quantities of hormones. Research has shown that nearly all the

women who have the symptoms of low thyroid have low tyrosine levels. It's also helpful in relieving depression on its own and as part of a thyroid treatment program. Tyrosine is found in meat, dairy, eggs, almonds, avocados, and bananas.

**Dosage:** Take up to 1,500 milligrams in divided doses each day.

**Side effects:** None known at this dosage; however, long-term effects of L-tyrosine in doses over 1,000 milligrams per day have not been studied.

**DHEA (dehydroepiandrosterone).** It's often called the "fountain of youth hormone" because DHEA can help you feel so much younger and more energetic. Japanese research shows people with hypothyroidism have less than 50 percent of the necessary levels of this hormone, which is essential for normal metabolism. "Hypothyroidism develops in part due to declining levels of DHEA as we age," says biochemist Stephen Cherniske, M.S., author of *The DHEA Breakthrough*. DHEA also helps your body produce estrogen and testosterone, so you should have a blood test to determine the correct amount for you to avoid too much of either of these sex hormones.

**Dosage:** Start at 5 milligrams a day and increase to not more than 10 milligrams.

**Side effects:** Can cause heart palpitations and arrhythmias at high doses. Do not exceed 10 milligrams per day and take "hormone holidays" at least a week every month.

---

### How to Take Thyroid Glandulars and L-Tyrosine

The same precautions apply to thyroid glandulars and L-tyrosine—take them on an empty stomach first thing in the morning at least three hours before your calcium- and iron-containing multivitamins for maximum absorption.

**Selenium.** Several studies have linked low levels of this mineral to thyroid malfunction. Recent research suggests that adding as little as 20 micrograms a day may bring your levels back to normal if the malfunction is due to a failure of thyroid hormones to activate properly.

"Everybody with a thyroid problem should be taking 200 micrograms of selenium a day," says Mary Shomon, author of *The Thyroid Diet.*

Note: Many good multivitamins already contain selenium, so check yours before adding a supplement.

**Dosage:** Up to 400 micrograms a day. Best taken with 400 IU of vitamin E.

**Side effects:** None known at this dosage.

**Iodine.** This mineral is essential for the production of thyroid hormones, but even though most of us use iodized salt, our iodine levels have dropped more than 50 percent in the past twenty years—a number that parallels the increase in thyroid disorders. While iodine supplementation is controversial, (see Chapter 1), there's no disagreement that we all need about 150 micrograms of iodine a day for thyroid health and to maintain breast health. Some practitioners think we get plenty from our food, especially iodized bread and salt.

**Dosage:** Consult with your doctor or healthcare practitioner. Dosage will depend on test results and the school of thought to which your caretaker subscribes. Most recommend supplementation in the neighborhood of 200 micrograms daily.

**Side effects:** Exceedingly high doses may impair thyroid function, causing either hypothyroidism or hyperthyroidism.

**Kelp, Bladderwrack, and Black Walnut.** These are natural sources of iodine often used to promote healthy glandular function by regulating the thyroid. Many people use them for thyroid deficiency, but Mary Shomon recommends caution in taking these since few Westerners are actually iodine deficient and a great deal of hypothyroidism found in the Western world is due to autoimmune disease that can be aggravated with excessive iodine supplementation. See the above section on iodine and Chapter 1, and consult your healthcare practitioner for dosages and precautions before taking any of these.

**Essential Fatty Acids, especially Evening Primrose Oil.** Essential fatty acids (omega-3, found in cold water fish and flaxseed; and omega-6, found in whole grains, eggs, poultry, and vegetable oils) are powerful antioxidants and among the most important promoters of overall health known to science. While all are important to general health, evening primrose oil has a particular connection to thyroid health. While reviewing the scientific research on the subject, Dr. Stephen Langer realized that evening primrose oil and thyroid hormones work on an almost identical list of symptoms.

Dr. Langer theorizes this is because the gamma-linolenic acid in evening primrose oil helps promote the body's natural production of prostaglandins, and like thyroid hormones, prostaglandins are involved in metabolism, blood circulation, growth and reproduction, and immune system function. "Individuals low in prostaglandins catch every communicable disease. So do hypothyroids," writes Dr. Langer in *Solved: The Riddle of Illness*.
**Dosage:** Up to 1,000 milligrams three times daily.
**Side effects:** Bloating and gastrointestinal upset in a small number of users.

**Coconut Oil.** Coconut oil has been touted as a "cure" for hypothyroidism, and while there's no scientific evidence to back that up, there is plenty of research that shows it stimulates metabolism, raises basal body temperatures, and boosts energy. It has been shown to be very helpful in promoting weight loss for some people, including those with hypothyroidism. Coconut oil is nature's best source of medium-chain fatty acids or MCFAs that immediately produce energy in your body, unlike other oils that are stored as fat until your body needs extra energy. In addition, researchers at Nashville's Vanderbilt University say eating coconut oil can increase your calorie burning power by 50 percent.

**Dosage:** Up to 3.5 tablespoons of extra virgin organically produced coconut oil daily. Warning: If you use it for frying, keep temperatures below 325°F.

**Side effects:** None known.

### *Energy Enhancers*

The following supplements can help boost your energy.

**Vitamin B Complex.** Flagging energy is probably one of the most common symptoms of hypothyroidism, so getting sufficient amounts of B vitamins essential for energy will help neutralize that problem. Vitamins $B_2$, $B_3$, and $B_6$ are part of the thyroxine production process. Vitamin $B_{12}$ is particularly important in the energy chain of hypothyroidism and $B_{12}$ supplementation is often recommended. If you are hypothyroid and feel tingling in the hands, feet, or face; have a low pulse rate or palpitations; try some $B_{12}$.

If your blood levels of $B_{12}$ have tested low (under 540 pg/mL), Dr. Teitelbaum recommends $B_{12}$ shots containing 3,000 micrograms of the vitamin three times a week for up to twenty treatments. If injections are not available, he recommends taking 1,000 to 5,000 micrograms a day in supplement form. Strict vegetarians and vegans will have $B_{12}$ deficiency unless they take supplements, since animal protein is the only known dietary source of $B_{12}$.

Find an enteric coated 5,000 microgram $B_{12}$ tablet, since $B_{12}$ is destroyed by stomach acid, the enteric coating prevents it from dissolving until it reaches the small intestine where it can be absorbed. Shomon recommends a sublingual $B_{12}$ for a quick and noticeable energy boost.

Dosage: This is a list of the B vitamins and the recommended dosages for adults. If you buy a B complex, the simplest way to get all of them, be sure it contains the following amounts:

| B vitamin | DRI* | Therapeutic Dosage** |
|---|---|---|
| $B_1$ (thiamine) | 1.5 mg | 50–250 mg |
| $B_2$ (riboflavin) | 1.7 mg | 10–200 mg |
| $B_3$ (niacin/niacinamide) | 15–20 mg | 50–100 mg |
| $B_5$ (pantothenic acid) | 10 mg | 250 mg–2 g |
| $B_6$ (pyridoxine) | 2.5 mg | 50–100 mg |
| $B_7$ (biotin) | 300 mcg | 15–1,000 mcg |
| $B_9$ (folic acid/folate) | 400 mcg–20 mg | 400–1,000 mcg |
| $B_{12}$ (hydroxyl) | 4–6 mcg | 50 mcg–10 mg |

Side effects: None known at DRI levels.

*DRI stands for Daily Reference Intakes

**You should work with a nutritionally oriented physician before supplementing at the higher ranges of the therapeutic dosages.

**Coenzyme $Q_{10}$.** Better known as $CoQ_{10}$, this enzyme helps you harvest the maximum energy from your food and thereby boost your energy levels. It also enhances immune function, assists in weight loss, and improves exercise tolerance because it supplies energy to the muscles. In addition, high thyroid function can actually burn the $CoQ_{10}$ out of your body at a very fast rate, resulting in heart failure, so $CoQ_{10}$ supplementation is essential if you have been diagnosed with hyperthyroidism.

It's also essential if you are taking any of the cholesterol-lowering statin drugs, such as Lipitor, Zocor, Pravachol, etc., for the same reasons. These drugs, meant to decrease the incidence of heart disease actually deplete the body's supply of $CoQ_{10}$ and can cause heart failure.

**Dosage:** Start with 30 to 50 milligrams per day and work your way to 100 milligrams daily or until you feel the increased energy effects. Many patients on statin drugs are advised to take 1 milligram per pound of body weight daily, so if you weigh 150 pounds, take 150 milligrams. $CoQ_{10}$ works best is taken with a little fat.

**Side effects:** High dosages can cause restlessness and insomnia. If these occur, reduce your dosage.

**Acetyl-L-Carnitine.** This amino acid helps transport fatty acids across cell membranes to create energy. It also helps burn fat, reduce depression and improve mental performance. Acetyl-L-carnitine is used for virtually every body function and low levels contribute to fatigue, muscle weakness, and cramping. Acetyl-L-carnitine is found primarily in red meats, so vegetarians often are deficient in this important nutrient and should consider supplementation.

**Dosage:** Take 300 milligrams up to 2 grams daily.

**Side effects:** Can cause increased blood pressure, so you should monitor your blood pressure if you are taking this supplement. At high doses, it can also cause an elevated heart rate and diarrhea.

**NADH (Nicotinamide Adenine Dinucleotide plus High Energy Hydrogen).** This coenzyme, made by your body from vitamin $B_3$ helps cells convert food into energy. NADH stimulates the production of ATP (adenosine triphosphate), a compound that regulates the release of energy stored in cells. The more NADH a cell has, the more chemical energy it produces, and therefore the more energy you have. Research shows NADH is helpful in relieving fatigue, even chronic fatigue and fibromyalgia, and in improving mental function, even in patients with Alzheimer's.

**Dosage:** Take two 5-milligram tablets every morning for six to twelve weeks. Dr. Teitelbaum recommends taking only the Enada brand of this supplement (the only one that won't be neutralized by stomach acid) first thing in the morning on an empty stomach and at least one-half hour before any other medications or supplements except thyroid hormones, if you are taking them. It may take up to three months to see results.

**Side effects:** Can cause restlessness and insomnia at high doses.

**Green Tea Extract.** Several studies have found that green tea and green tea extract will speed up metabolic rates beyond the increase that would be expected because of its caffeine content alone. While some studies show a small increase in calorie burning with green tea, scientists have found that the extra expenditure took place during the daytime. According to Shormon, this led researchers to conclude that, since thermogenesis (the body's own rate of burning calories) contributes 8–10 percent of daily energy expenditure in a typical subject, that this 4 percent overall increase in energy expenditure due to the green tea actually translated to a 35–43 percent increase in daytime thermogenesis. So, green tea will help increase energy and help with weight loss issues that affect most people with hypothyroidism.

**Dosage:** Drink three to five cups of green tea daily or take 250-500 milligrams daily.

**Side effects:** None known at recommended dosage.

**Panax Ginseng (also known as Korean or Asian Ginseng).** This adaptogenic herb supports the body's capacity for work. Some studies also suggest that ginseng may also reduce the release of the stress hormone cortisol by the adrenals and stop damage to the adrenals and the thyroid. Panax ginseng may be too stimulating for some people.

**Dosage:** Up to 600 milligrams in divided doses daily. Some sources recommend a one-week "holiday" every two to three months.

**Side effects:** Not recommended for people with

high blood pressure. Can cause restlessness, headaches, and diarrhea.

**Mate tea.** Yerba mate, pronounced, "mah-tay," is
an energizing herbal tea that is hugely popular in
South America, where it is considered a healthy
alternative to coffee. Mate is a rich source of antioxidants and has many of the same nutritional con-
stituents found in green tea (but it has a very
different and acquired taste). It also has some caffeine, roughly half the amount found in a serving of
coffee, but aficionados say its effects are energizing, rather than making people jittery.
**Dosage:** One to three cups a day.
**Side effects:** Yerba mate has been reported to have
MAO-inhibitor activity in one in vitro study. If you're
taking MAO-inhibitor drugs for depression, you
should use yerba mate with caution.

### Combination supplements
Combination supplements can be very helpful in
promoting thyroid function. Some of the best are
discussed below.

**Energy Revitalization.** Energy revitalization, based
on Dr. Teitelbaum's research, is a powder that can
be mixed with water, milk, yogurt, or fruit drinks. It
contains several amino acids including L-tyrosine
and several dozen other ingredients designed to
help raise energy levels. It's available at most health
food stores.
**Dosage:** $1/2$ to 1 scoop daily along with the recommended B-complex capsule.
**Side effects:** Diarrhea occurs occasionally. Can be
counteracted by starting at a low dosage and grad-
ually working up to a dosage that feels best.

**Padma Basic.** Padma Basic is a formulation based
on the principles of traditional Chinese medicine
and is highly recommended by Drs. Shames to nor-
malize immune function and particularly to help

overcome the autoimmune deficiency that can cause Hashimoto's hypothyroidism. It contains, among other herbs, Iceland moss, costus root, and neem fruit. Padma Basic is available over the counter at better health food stores.

**Dosage:** Take two tablets a day according to manufacturer's instructions.

**Side effects:** None known at recommended dosage.

**Thyro-Sense.** This blend of nutrients includes L-tyrosine, pantothenic acid, iodine, copper, ashwagandha, and guggul. It brings thyroid treatment modalities in the East and West together. These herbs and supplements are among the most effective natural treatments used in Western natural medicine and the ones most often used in Indian Ayurvedic medicine. The ingredients appear to have synergistic effects. Thyro-Sense can be taken alone or with thyroid hormone replacement to enhance its effects. This supplement is sold under numerous brand names.

**Dosage:** Take up to four capsules daily in divided doses; it can be taken at the same time you take your thyroid hormone pills. Take other supplements at a different time.

**Side effects:** None known at recommended dosage.

### *Other Natural Modalities*

If you haven't already done so, take the opportunity now to try yoga, tai chi, or chi gong. These Eastern disciplines are all excellent means of adding and balancing energy to your body, mind, and spirit. In chi gong, tai chi, and yoga, slow, gentle movements help move energy along the energy pathways of the body, resulting in better balance for all body systems. Chi gong is a Chinese system of prescribed physical exercises or movements performed in a meditative state. Tai chi is a traditional Chinese mind-body relaxation exercise consisting of 108 intricate exercise sequences performed in a slow, relaxed manner over a thirty-minute period.

Yoga is an ancient Indian discipline that includes asanas (specific physical movements), breathing exercises, meditation, and relaxation. One particular yoga posture, the Shoulder Stand (or sarvangasana, literally translated as the "do-everything" posture) is excellent for stimulating thyroid function because you are upside down with your chin tucked into your jugular notch, stimulating the thyroid.

If you're considering any of these forms of wellness and relaxation, I highly recommend taking at least one course from a qualified instructor to learn the proper forms and to prevent injury.

### Adrenal Support

If tests show you have impaired adrenal function, supplementation with DHEA and/or Panax ginseng can help improve adrenal function. See discussion earlier in this chapter about these supplements.

In addition, you may find the following helpful.

**Adrenal Glandular.** These supplements can help address the fatigue, stress, and infections often associated with toxic stress. Glandular preparations, usually made from the adrenal glands of cattle, work in much the same way as desiccated thyroid hormones. For a high quality over-the-counter preparation, Drs. Shames recommend IsoCort, containing standardized quantities of the glandular hormones, including hydrocortisone. There are also liquid forms and homeopathic remedies. If you decide to take a homeopathic, Drs. Shames recommend taking it for not more than three weeks, then allowing your body to find its own balance, as is intended with homeopathics.

**Dosage:** Take according to manufacturer's instructions.

**Side effects:** None known at recommended dosage.

## Hyperthyroidism

Testing for DHEA levels is recommended for those with hyperthyroidism.

Some people get positive results from adding fluoride (under the direction of your health-care practitioner), selenium, or copper (see discussion earlier in this chapter).

**Motherwort.** This herb, which grows wild throughout much of the United States and Canada, has been approved by the German Commission E (the equivalent of the American FDA) as part of the treatment for hyperthyroidism and can relieve heart palpitations. Motherwort is available in the United States in several preparations, among them a good quality extract manufactured by Gaia Herbs.
**Dosage:** Use according to manufacturer's instructions.
**Side effects:** None known.

# CHAPTER 9

# DIETARY APPROACHES AND WEIGHT LOSS

Other than eating a generally healthy diet rich in fruits and vegetables, lean meats, healthy fats, and lots of water, there aren't specific dietary recommendations to keep your thyroid hormones balanced. However, some foods, generally considered healthy, can be harmful to some people with very sensitive thyroids when eaten raw and in large quantities. These foods, called "goitrogens" include cruciferous vegetables such as broccoli, Brussels sprouts, cauliflower, and cabbage. Cooking neutralizes the harmful effects, so this is usually not a problem for those with hypothyroidism unless you consume large quantites of them in raw form every day. A serving of coleslaw does not a goiter make.

## The Soy Controversy

Some controversial research suggests that overconsumption of soy products may trigger an autoimmune response in sensitive people.

Again, we're not talking about a veggie burger here and there, we're talking about the folks Mary Shomon calls "soy crazy"—of the if-some-is-good-more-is-better school.

"What you don't want to be doing are soy smoothies for breakfast, soy powders for snacks, soy nuts, burgers, creams all day long. If you are going to eat soy, eat it in moderation and use it in its natural form like the Asians. That means tempeh or tofu, not pills powders and shakes. Edamame is fine in reasonable quantities as well, for most people," says Shomon.

## Weight Control

Hypothyroidism and overweight almost always go hand-in-hand. The lowered metabolic rate associated with hypothyroidism makes it difficult, if not impossible, for most sufferers to lose weight. That's why Dr. Sanford Siegal devised the draconian 1,000-calorie diet plan to diagnose low thyroid function. As he says, "If you don't lose weight or don't lose as much weight as a 'normal' person on this plan, we know you have a thyroid problem." A 1,000-calorie diet is a difficult challenge—and it's one most of us aren't up to.

You're probably sick to death of doctors telling you that the key to weight loss is to do "pushaways" from the dinner table and get off your lard butt and take a brisk walk once a day. I know all of you wish it were that simple. You know as well as I do, it's not simple at all. And worst of all, many people who do finally get diagnosed and get on the right medication find they still don't lose weight for reasons no one really understands.

This isn't a diet book, and I'm not going to go into great detail about diet here, but I'm going to quickly throw out some ideas from Mary Shomon, author of *The Thyroid Diet*. You can go more deeply into these if you wish. Shomon thinks our bodies know what they need—and everyone's body is different, so the weight loss plan that works for your best friend won't necessarily work for you, let alone for your co-worker or your sister. Each of us is biologically unique.

Shomon has devised different diet plans for people with a variety of diet challenges, ranging from those who have gained weight on Atkins, South Beach, and/or Weight Watchers; to those who feel they eat too much and are unable to stop; to those who gain weight even if they've cut back on portions and fattening foods.

She boils them down to two types: the Free Form Eater and the Carbohydrate-Sensitive Eater, and offers a four-week plan to help you figure out which you are and which works best for you. In the simplest possible terms, the Free Form Eater is encouraged to eat a relatively high protein, low glycemic index diet, with lots of water and fiber and very little fruit or other sweets. The Carbohydrate Sensitive type eats fewer carbohydrates, more vegetables, less fruit, and more fiber.

# CONCLUSION

I know there's literally a lot to swallow here in this short book, so take your time with it, digest it, and take what works for you. I also know it can be overwhelming to try to cope with hypothyroidism and its seemingly endless variety of accompanying problems. Stick with your search, no matter how discouraging it may be to find a diagnosis or the right treatment. Use the resources here and become a bulldog about it—don't let go until you get the treatment you need and want.

You do not have to be old before your time. You don't have to sit on life's sidelines, watching others have fun. Good health, high energy, and a long life are your birthright. Claim them.

# OTHER BOOKS
# AND RESOURCES

Ahlgrimm, Marla, and Kells, John M. *The HRT Solution* (Avery, 1999).

Barnes, Kathleen. *User's Guide to Natural Hormone Replacement* (Basic Health Publications, 2005).

Blumenthal M., ed. *The Complete German Commission E Monographs: Therapeutic Guide to Herbal Medicines.* Boston, Mass: Integrative Medicine Communications, 1998.

Brownstein, David. *Iodine, Why You Need It, Why You Can't Live without It* (available through his website, www.drbrownstein.com).

Cass, Hyla, and Barnes, Kathleen. *8 Weeks to Vibrant Health* (McGraw-Hill, 2004).

Langer, Stephen, and Scheer, James. *Solved: The Riddle of Illness* (Keats, 2000).

Moore, Elaine and Lisa. *Graves' Disease: A Practical Guide* (McFarland and Co., 2001).

Shames, Richard L., and Shames, Karilee. *Thyroid Power* (Quill, 2002).

Shomon, Mary. *Living Well with Hypothyroidism* (Quill, 2005).

Shomon, Mary. *The Thyroid Diet* (Harper Collins, 2004).

Siegal, Sanford. *Is Your Thyroid Making You Fat?* (Warner Books, 2000).

Teitelbaum, Jacob. *From Fatigued to Fantastic* (Avery, 2001).

## To find the best doctors for thyroid disorders:

Mary Shomon's Thyroid Top Doctors Directory:
www.thyroid-info.com/topdrs

Armour thyroid/Thyrolar doctor database:
www.armourthyroid.com/locate.html

American Osteopathic Association:
www.aoa-net.org

American Holistic Medical Association:
www.holisticmedicine.org

## Websites:

Broda Barnes Foundation:
www.brodabarnes.org

Mary Shomon's thyroid website:
www.thyroid.about.com

Dr. Jacob Teitelbaum's website:
www.vitality101.com

Thyroid Foundation of America:
www.allthyroid.org

Kripalu Yoga Centers:
www.kripalu.org
(In my mind, the best yoga teachers around.)

## Magazines:

### GreatLife Magazine
Consumer magazine with articles on vitamins, minerals, herbs, and foods.
*Available for free at many health and natural food stores.*

### Let's Live Magazine
Consumer magazine with emphasis on the health benefits of vitamins, minerals, and herbs.
**Customer service:**
1-800-676-4333
P.O. Box 74908
Los Angeles, CA 90004
*Subscriptions: 12 issues per year, $19.95 in the U.S.;
$31.95 outside the U.S.*

### Physical Magazine

Magazine oriented to body builders and other serious athletes.

**Customer service:**
1-800-676-4333
P.O. Box 74908
Los Angeles, CA 90004
*Subscriptions: 12 issues per year, $19.95 in the U.S.;*
*$31.95 outside the U.S.*

### The Nutrition Reporter™ newsletter

Monthly newsletter that summarizes recent medical research on vitamins, minerals, and herbs.

**Customer service:**
P.O. Box 30246
Tucson, AZ 85751-0246
e-mail: jack@thenutritionreporter.com
www.nutritionreporter.com
*Subscriptions: $26 per year (12 issues) in the U.S.; $32 U.S.*
*or $48 CNC for Canada; $38 for other countries*

# SELECTED
# REFERENCES

American Association of Clinical Endocrinologists. "Thyroid hormone missing from menopause discussion for millions of women." News release, January 13, 1999.

Adline, V. "Subclinical hypothyroidism: Deciding when to treat." *American Family Practice Magazine*, February 15, 1998 (online edition).

Bunevicius, R., Kazanavicius, Z., Zalinkevicius, R., et al. "Effects of thyroxine as compared with thyroxine plus triiodothyronine in patients with hypothyroidism." *New England Journal of Medicine*, 1999; 340(6): 424–429.

Gaby A.R. "Sub-laboratory hypothyroidism and the empirical use of Armour thyroid." *Alternative Medicine Review*. 2004; 9(2):157–179.

Jackson, A.S. "Hypothyroidism." *Journal of the American Medical Association* 1957, Sep 14; 165(2): 121–124.

Lowe, J.C. "Thyroid status of 38 fibromyalgia patients: Implications for the etiology of fibromyalgia." *Clinical Bulletin of Myofascial Therapy*, 1997; 2(1):47–64.

Mabuchi, H., Higasawa, T., Kawashiri, M., et al. "Reduction of serum ubiquinol-10 and ubiquinone-10 levels by atorvastatin in hypercholesterolemic patients." *Journal of Atherosclerosis and Thrombosis* 2005; 12(2):111–119.

Muller, B., Zulewski, H., Huber, P., et al. "Impaired action of thyroid hormone associated with smoking in women with hypothyroidism." *New England Journal of Medicine*, 1995; 333(15):1001–1002.

# INDEX

Printed in the USA
CPSIA information can be obtained
at www.ICGtesting.com
JSHW051956150824
68134JS00050B/70